Vesta Boyer
Bought   4-16-05
From   Library

Read -   4- 20-05 - Good Book

W9-AJQ-449

Not Quite a Miracle

Also by Jon Franklin and Alan Doelp
SHOCKTRAUMA

NOT QUITE A MIRACLE

Brain Surgeons and Their Patients on the Frontier of Medicine

Jon Franklin and Alan Doelp

HEMPHILL CO. LIBRARY
CANADIAN, TEXAS 79014

30,008

Doubleday & Company, Inc., Garden City, New York
1983

TEXAS STATE LIBRARY
FIELD SERVICES DIVISION
AUSTIN, TEXAS 78711
ON PERMANENT LOAN TO
CANADIAN PUBLIC LIBRARY

Library of Congress Cataloging in Publication Data

Franklin, Jon.
    Not quite a miracle.

    Includes index.
    1. Brain—Surgery.   2. Neurosurgeons.
3. Physician and patient.   I. Doelp, Alan.
II. Title.
RD594.F73   1983   617'.481
ISBN: 0-385-17495-0
Library of Congress Catalog Card Number 82–45461

Copyright © 1983 by Jon Franklin and Alan Doelp

All Rights Reserved
Printed in the United States of America
First Edition

In Memory of Edna Kelly
1921–1978

"Don't ever pull on anything. Not ever. You don't know what it's attached to. It might be attached to something that's attached to something that's attached to the soul."

—Michael Salcman, M.D.

ACKNOWLEDGMENTS

We owe substantial gratitude to the patients and family members who, despite their desperate circumstances, took time to tell us their stories. Their willingness to share their experiences with us testifies to the basic openness of the human spirit. Though several were dying, not one patient that we approached refused to talk to us.

We are repaying part of our debt to two of those families by changing their names and altering their circumstances enough to ensure their anonymity while remaining faithful to their stories. Except for them (and Joe Trott's resident, who is an amalgam of all the harried residents we watched) the stories you are about to read are true. The names are real names. The events we describe we either witnessed personally or researched and documented in exhaustive detail.

We took special pains to make the book accurate in context as well as fact. Our aim was more than just to tell stories; we wanted to give the reader a perception of what it is like to enter the operating room, what it is like to be a brain surgeon, what it is like to sit on the edge of your bed the night before the operation and think about what the morning will bring.

Each patient expressed the hope that this book would prove valuable to other brain surgery patients and their families. We share that sentiment, most particularly because the message, for the first time in the history of neurosurgery, is a positive one. Brain surgery remains a gamble, but the odds are better now than ever before.

This larger story could not have been told without the co-operation of the many neurosurgeons, neurologists, neuroanatomists, neurochemists and neuroscientists we interviewed at both the University of Maryland and Johns Hopkins medical schools. They took time out of busy schedules to talk to us, to explain the function of the brain to us and, when we didn't understand the first time, to patiently explain it again. These superb teachers not only train future generations of doctors and scientists, they also provide the basis for public understanding of medical science, and they have our respect and gratitude.

This book is about the enduring courage of brain surgery patients, but it owes its existence to a much more subtle courage on the part of four brain surgeons: Dr. Tom Ducker and Dr. Michael Salcman at the University of Maryland Hospital and Dr. Donlin Long and Dr. Kenneth Murray at Johns Hopkins. They allowed us to enter what traditionally has been a very private world.

In being open, and in allowing us to portray them as they are, they admit to their humanity—and fallibility. No doubt they will be criticized by some of their colleagues for their candor, but we believe their experiences, honestly told, will bring honor to their profession and understanding to their patients.

We also owe a special gratitude to Dr. Marshall Rennels and Dr. George Samaras. Dr. Rennels patiently tutored us in neuroanatomy and, when we could absorb no more, in sailing. Dr. Samaras taught us enough engineering to understand the finicky Capricorn machine.

In addition we would thank those many doctors and scientists who contributed to our project but whose names, in the end, appear only fleetingly (if at all) in the book. They include Dr. Richard T. Johnson, Dr. Hamilton Moses, Dr. Michael Kuhar, Dr. Solomon Snyder, Dr. Candace Pert, Dr. John Freeman, Dr. Nathan Schnaper, Dr. Tom Price, Dr. Jane Matjasko, Dr. Nelson Hendler, Dr. John Rybock, Dr. Walker Robinson, Dr. Ron Cohen, Dr. Hatem Abdo, Dr. Gary Magram, Dr. Ernesto Botero, Dr. Miguel Machado, Dr. Sylvain Palmer, Dr. Daniel Heffez and Dr. Thomas Sanchez.

We are particularly grateful to the nurses and technicians who coped with our presence in the operating rooms, and who always had time to stop and, in a few hurried phrases, explain what was going on. This book would have been poorer without the help of people like Kay Donnelly, Doris Schwabland, Willie House and Sharon Land. Also, our thanks to Mary Cooper, the nurse in charge of the Johns Hopkins Pain Treatment Center.

Because this book is focused on the patients, the influence of the surgeons' wives, families and home lives did not get the attention it deserved. But Barbara Ducker, Harriet Long, Sandra Murray and Ilene Salcman are very real, very wonderful women whose depth of understanding and unceasing good-naturedness have contributed in no small measure to their husbands' success.

Nor can we overlook the very important role of the surgeons' secretaries. Organizing a neurosurgeon's schedule is a job of epic proportions, but Barbara Burns, Fran Crow, Pat Diniar and Sharon Wellslager made it look simple, and they handled our erratic, often panic-stricken phone calls with unfailing courtesy and competence. It is possible that we could have written the book without their help, but we'd hate to try.

In the world of New York, in which authors are functional innocents, we relied on the sensitive counsel of Adrian Zackheim, our editor at Doubleday, and on the early encouragement of Denis Holler, our agent.

In the writing of this book we also benefited from the patience and advice of our friends and families. We would like to especially acknowledge the literary aid and comfort provided by Lynn Scheidhauer and Cathy Franklin.

We wrote and rewrote the manuscript for this book on a pair of very excellent Compucorp word processors, an experience that makes us wonder how we ever got by with mere typewriters. We are grateful to Bob Bogar, Chuck Cavolo, and Mark Zutkoff for all their good advice and cybernetic hand-holding.

A special thanks also to Dana Levitz, who periodically read our copy and reassured us that we were better than Shakespeare. There were dark days when we needed that. Also to Kelly Gilbert, who read our copy and pointed out, in sobering detail, that Dana was somewhat . . . well, generous. Alas, we needed that even more.

Writing a book is a growth experience, and one of the many lessons we both learned was that . . . something . . . can . . . always . . . happen.

As Tom Ducker likes to say, neurosurgeons don't walk on water. Neither do authors who write about them. Nothing is perfect, including this book. We must share much of the credit for its merits, but the errors are our responsibility, and ours alone.

Jon Franklin
Alan Doelp
Baltimore, 1982

Not Quite a Miracle

CHAPTER
ONE

THE BROWN OLDSMOBILE MOVED DOWN THE LOOP DRIVE, BENEATH RIS-
ing cliffs of brick and steel, and came to a stop in front of the lobby of
Johns Hopkins Hospital. The rear door opened and a slight young
man slowly emerged into the frigid Baltimore weather, tottered
slightly, and leaned on the car. A security guard stepped forward to
steady him, but the young man motioned him away.

No, he did not want a wheelchair. Definitely not.

He let the car door go and walked unsteadily toward the automatic
glass doors. The Oldsmobile pulled out and nosed into the traffic on
Wolfe Street, heading toward the parking lot.

The young man made his way slowly and carefully across the warm
lobby, past the tropical palms that grew in knee-high decorator pots.
Broad-leafed foliage hung over the mezzanine railing.

The tumor had caused his eyes to point in different directions,
causing double vision, so he had to close one of them in order to locate
the open door marked ADMITTING. In the admitting office he
waited his turn at the reception counter, gave his name, accepted a
form letter, and sat down in a soft orange chair. In a few minutes his
mother and father, having parked the Oldsmobile, joined him.

He squinted at the letter. It cheerfully explained that a hospital like
the Hopkins needed to know a great deal about its patients, which
meant interviews and tests. He passed the letter to his mother, settled
back, and closed both eyes. In a few minutes a woman ushered the
three of them into a small room to talk about insurance.

After the woman had filled out the forms, and his father had signed
them, his parents were sent back to the lobby. Another hospital
worker fastened a plastic band around the new patient's wrist. The patient held the wristband up to his right eye. Ah. Now he had a number.

Eventually a nurse came to draw a vial of blood from Case No.

191-00-18's arm, then sent him on to yet another room to wait his turn for a chest X-ray. Finally they offered him a wheelchair for the trip to his room.

No.

No wheelchair.

No way.

A half hour later he sat on the edge of a tautly made bed, listening to the escort's footsteps fade away down the hallway. Then he looked again at the wristband. The plastic was also stamped with the name of the admitting physician, a Dr. Ronald Cohen—the chief resident in neurosurgery. Like every other brain surgeon the young man had met recently, Dr. Cohen was fascinated by his X-rays.

Case No. 191-00-18 bounced thoughtfully on the bed. In the last few days he'd learned enough about medicine to know that when the doctors got interested, that was not good.

A nurse came in, assured herself that all was well, and offered to help him undress. She accepted his refusal cheerfully. Later, his parents came up, fidgeted awhile, then went home. The nurse brought a sleeping pill, but he declined it. On the way out she turned off the light. He lay quietly on the bed, listening to the sounds of the hospital.

The next morning an escort came for him with a wheelchair. Case No. 191-00-18 sat up in the bed and looked at the thing. Chrome and spokes glinted back at him.

No, he said. No wheelchair.

The escort was friendly, reasonable.

Look, man. Everybody rides the wheelchair. You'll get a lot more stares if you try to walk. Who ever heard of letting a patient walk? Are you trying to put me out of a job?

The patient didn't consent graciously but he consented, and for the next few days he allowed himself to be pushed slowly from one part of the hospital to another and parked unceremoniously in public hallways outside closed doors. At first he tried to read, but it was difficult to keep one eye closed and the other open. Soon he, like the other patients, just sat there, woolgathering, too polite to stare at the others, too listless to attempt conversation.

As time passed, each of the patients in turn would be called into the room and the door closed. In a few minutes that person was wheeled out and down the hall. The waiting patients scrutinized him as he went by, and then another would be called, and the door closed again. Finally Case No. 191-00-18 would progress from newcomer to first in line, and they would push him through the door.

Sometimes they just looked in his eyes, or made him listen to clicks and whistles. Sometimes they made him stand or sit in awkward positions, and other times they stuck him with pins. Once he lay on a table staring straight up while some sort of camera-head or imager rotated above him on an oval track, stopped periodically and emitted loud clicks.

Another time they laid him on a table, pointed an X-ray device at his head, stuck a needle into the inside of his thigh and injected something into his veins. The something felt like molten steel, and Case No. 191-00-18 stifled a cry. His head exploded and the camera clicked, and then they put him back in the wheelchair and trundled him off for the next test.

Case No. 191-00-18 understood some of the tests, had vague notions about some others, and was completely baffled by a few. But the most important test of all was the CAT scan, and it was also the most interesting. As it was explained to him, the CAT-scanner shot an X-ray beam through the head, fed the information into a computer and reconstructed whatever view of the brain the doctor wanted. From where he sat, waiting, he could see the thing through an open door. He could even glimpse an image of someone else's brain hanging in the center of a computer screen.

Fascinating. Now what kind of program would it take, he wondered, to turn a string of electronic pulses into an image that looked just like a slice of a living brain? No longer bored, he combed his knowledge of mathematics and computing.

A digital-imaging algorithm, he finally concluded. Relatively simple. The same sort of gimmick NASA uses to reconstruct pictures of Saturn.

When it was his turn, they rolled him into the room and let him climb from the wheelchair onto a long wooden table that lay in front of what appeared to be a giant steel doughnut. He lay with his head toward the doughnut hole, like an Aztec sacrifice at the gaping mouth of a stone god. The god's name was Pfizer, to judge by the raised-metal lettering.

One wall of the room was dominated by a series of glass windows, through which the patient could watch the technicians hunched over their computer terminals. He closed one eye, resolving the face of a pretty young technician who watched him, thoughtfully, through the curling smoke of a cigarette. One of the men who had brought him in told him to lie very still. Then everyone left the room and someone closed the door.

The table moved, and his head slid into the huge doughnut hole. There was a smell of light oil. Case No. 191-00-18 closed his eyes.

Beyond the lead glass, the woman laid the cigarette in an ashtray and touched a button. Lights flickered across the consoles. The faint whir of a servomotor vibrated through the metallic wall and an image appeared on the screen.

Ding went a bell, announcing the completion of the first image.

The scanner operator glanced down at the screen, up at the patient, and back down at the screen, assuring herself that all was in order.

The first slice was through the crown of the skull, catching just the tops of the two hemispheres. Two small half-circles of brain, surrounded by a ring of skull, glowed on the screen.

The image was technically excellent. The woman touched several keys, and the lights flashed faster than before.

Ding.

The second image was similar to the first, but the circle was bigger.

Ding.

As the slices cut deeper into the brain, a small black spot appeared at the center of each hemisphere. These represented the main ventricles of the brain, the central caverns where cerebral spinal fluid is manufactured and stored.

The technician frowned as the black spots enlarged with each slice. They were perceptibly larger than normal.

Ding.

Beyond the lead glass, the doughnut hummed and clicked and the table advanced. The pulses of information streamed into the computer's core, where they were arranged into a map. With each image the patient's head moved a fraction of an inch farther into the doughnut hole.

The technician's eyes scanned the console, flitted across the screen and came to rest again on the patient. Another technician appeared behind her, looking at the slices.

Ding.

Ding.

Ding.

The machine buzzed, clicked and whined.

Ding.

Ding.

The ventricles were definitely enlarged. With a wave of his arm, the second technician summoned a third.

See, the second technician said, pointing the blunt tip of a ball-point pen at the screen. Something has blocked the drainage from the high ventricles and the cerebral spinal fluid has backed up, causing the ventricles to swell outward and push against the brain tissue. Since the brain and the ventricles are enclosed inside the skull with no way to expand, the pressure in the boy's head must be very high.

The third technician, a young man with an almost invisible blond mustache, listened soberly to the explanation. The machine whirred, dinged and cut deeper, approaching the level of the ears. As slice replaced slice, the enlarged ventricles disappeared and the complex structures of the lower brain came into view.

The junior technician stared at the succession of slices. The deep brain structures seemed out of place. He asked a question, but the senior man, engrossed, stared at the screen without answering.

Ding.

Ding.

Ding.

The brain narrowed at the bottom of the skull and then, when the patient's head had disappeared entirely into the doughnut, the console lights stopped flashing. The woman pushed another button and most of the lights winked out. The two male technicians left the booth and entered the scanner room.

One more, they told the patient. Only this time, they would use a chemical contrast medium.

Case No. 191-00-18 watched as the younger man handed a hypodermic needle to the older one. The patient winced slightly as the needle penetrated the skin of his arm. This time, the chemical didn't feel like molten metal. It hardly hurt at all.

The men left the room. The doughnut clicked. A motor hummed as the table moved. The woman watched through the thick, radiation-proof glass as the patient's head slowly disappeared into the scanner.

Afterward, Case No. 191-00-18 climbed off the table and into a wheelchair. The younger of the two technicians pushed the chair outside, parked it in the hallway, and reassured the boy that the metallic taste in his mouth was a side effect of the contrast medium—and warned him that the other side effect was an increased and urgent need to urinate as the body flushed the alien substance out through the kidneys.

The technician wheeled the next case into the scanner room and then placed a call to the escort service. In fifteen minutes or so, Case No. 191-00-18 should be waiting outside someone else's door.

In the CAT-scanner control center, the computer sorted and rearranged the data points that corresponded to the various structures inside Case No. 191-00-18's brain. Finally, it filed them so that, at the touch of a button, the patient's surgeon, Dr. Kenneth Murray, could order any slice he wanted to see.

As a matter of course, the scanner chief directed his crew to print a number of images on X-ray film. You could look at the images on the scanner screen, but the negatives were clearer. Besides, the docs were used to looking at negatives on lightboards.

In his years in big hospitals, the scanner chief had come to respect the impact of habit on the medical profession. Docs had to make a thousand little decisions a day and they had their routines. Routines become habit over the years. And breaking a habit was an uncomfortable thing to do.

Back in the electronic dark ages twenty yeas ago, docs looked at X-ray negatives because X-ray machines produced images on negative film. Today, when they could get their data in a rainbow of colors if they wanted, the docs were still most comfortable with negatives. Ironically, that meant technicians had to have special equipment specifically to transfer the data from the memory banks to an archaic medium—photographic film.

In his years in medical technology the chief technician had learned a great deal about what the docs were looking for, and why. Now it wasn't unusual at all for him to offer a suggestion, when it was needed. By the time the doc came out of the room, he usually remembered it as being his own idea.

The technician thought about the scans on No. 191-00-18. Some cases were dull, and some were interesting; some were *very* interesting, and some . . .

He would make some extra copies. If he knew anything about docs at all, they would want to pass this one around.

The case belonged to Dr. Kenneth Murray, a neurosurgeon who also had a PhD in tumor immunology. For more than a decade he had worked closely with the chairman of neurosurgery, Dr. Donlin Long. He was Dr. Long's expert on tumors.

And, the technician observed, this kid was sorely in need of a tumor specialist.

When the data in the CAT-scan computer had been reduced to images on film, they were sent to Dr. Murray. He pulled them out of the yellow envelope and snapped them under the lightboard clips. His eyes went instantly to the slices that showed the tumor's image, nestled against the brain stem.

He looked at the scans for several minutes, then stuck his head through the door of Dr. John Rybock's office, next door. A few moments later both doctors stood in front of the X-ray board. Dr. Rybock whistled appreciatively. No, he'd never seen one like that either.

The conversation attracted a third neurosurgeon, then a passing radiologist, then a medical secretary. Peering over a surgeon's shoulder, she could see instantly what the fuss was about. A posterior fossa tumor.

The posterior fossa is a compartment the size of a tennis ball, at the bottom of the brain where the spinal cord emerges into the cranium and expands to become the brain stem. The cavity is protected on the top by a tent of tough membranes and on the bottom by the floor of the skull.

In the course of evolution, the posterior fossa was shaped to cradle and protect the most delicate structures in nature, the processing centers of the brain stem. It is there that breathing, heartbeat and hormones are regulated, and where the higher centers are controlled. The brain stem is the pilot light of life and consciousness.

The brain specialists clustered around Case No. 191-00-18's CAT scans, talking excitedly in words that, among them, only the secretary had the ability to spell. The secretary couldn't follow the fine points of the discussion, but even she could see that the tumor was wrapped around the brain stem. The thing was huge.

"Huge" is a relative term. In the brain, where the basic processing and memory unit is microscopic, a growth the size of a walnut, like this one, was enough to make a medical secretary's eyes get wide.

In addition to damaging the brain centers it touched, the tumor's bulk would crowd the contents of the skull and, by raising the pressure, squeeze every center in the head. Even worse, if the tumor was in the posterior fossa it could block the drainage of spinal fluid, and make the pressure rise a little more. The combined pressures would make the entire brain swell, and that would increase the pressure further.

He could walk, the patient record said. The neurosurgeons shook their heads. He actually walked into the hospital alone.

Walked.

The doctors gazed at the scans and thought about it. Later, Dr. Murray went over the records again, and made the first of a long list of critical decisions. Dr. Long, he decided, would want to see this.

He put the negatives back into the envelope and walked out into the austere hallway. Two doors down, beyond the stairs to the neurosurgical library, he turned into Dr. Long's outer office.

Pat Diniar and Fran Crow, the secretaries, were both on the telephone. Dr. Murray waved at them and approached the chief neurosurgeon's door. He paused there until Dr. Long looked up from the couch. The chief laid aside the scientific paper he was reading and rose to his feet.

Dr. Murray said little, beyond a greeting. The scans told the story more eloquently. He turned on the lightboard and snapped the negatives into place. Dr. Long gazed at them, his hands in the pockets of his white coat.

Walked, huh?

Wow.

By now, of course, the patient was in a wheelchair. Dr. Murray had seen to that. Case No. 191-00-18 was being dealt with like an incipient disaster, which he was.

It might take only a sneeze, or an odd movement, or a bump on the head. Then Case No. 191-00-18's brain would shift slightly, easing the pressure. In the posterior fossa, a little bit of the cerebellum would deform, bend the brain stem and press against the top of the spinal cord. The movement would help lower the pressure in the brain, but the relief would be of little value to Case No. 191-00-18. The instant the brain stem shifted, that would be the end of, of, of . . .

Dr. Long looked at the name on the chart.

. . . the end of one Joseph T. Trott.

The chief neurosurgeon gazed at the tumor some more. By its location and staining characteristics, it was either a meningioma or an acoustic tumor. Either way, it was the biggest he had ever seen. And the boy was only twenty.

Dr. Long listened to Dr. Murray recite the patient's history, but his eyes stayed on the CAT scan.

Walked!

Wow.

CHAPTER

TWO

Dr. Thomas B. Ducker lay still beneath the warm blankets and let the chemicals of consciousness flow slowly through his brain. It was still night, and the alarm clock hadn't gone off yet. On mornings when he was scheduled to operate, it rarely got the chance.

Outside, the wind was howling through the branches of the oak trees. Was it snowing? The weatherman had said it might. The blankets were very warm.

Lazily, the neurosurgeon nudged his mind toward the day ahead. Josh. The eleven-year-old boy who couldn't play baseball.

He had stood in the center of the office, dressed in shined shoes, sharply creased slacks and a blue blazer. He looked Dr. Ducker directly in the eye. Could Dr. Ducker please fix it so he could play baseball again?

Dr. Ducker knelt on the carpet and helped the boy roll up his sleeve. The scar was on the inside of his right arm, halfway between elbow and armpit.

The neurosurgeon ran his fingers over the arm, expertly testing the tissue beneath. He had seen many like it before, during the Vietnam war, except that this scar was clean and narrow. Chunks of shrapnel are messy.

Dr. Ducker looked at the boy's numb fingers. He spread them apart, extending the curled hand. One by one, he examined each finger. The boy watched intently.

Baseball, huh?

First base, sir.

When he was Josh's age, Dr. Ducker said, he hadn't played much baseball. Soccer was more his game. Still. He could sympathize. Getting sidelined is miserable, whatever the sport.

Yes sir, said Josh.

Dr. Ducker got to his feet, conscious of the boy's eyes on his face.

He hesitated a moment as his mind digested the feel of the scar. He had read the boy's record earlier, and he knew the whole story.

Josh had run into a window, and a piece of the glass had fallen like a guillotine. It cut through the brachial artery, so the first efforts in the emergency room had been to stop him from bleeding to death. After that they called in a local neurosurgeon to look for severed nerves.

The neurosurgeon explored the wound, found the ends of the median nerve, and carefully sewed them together. Since nerves are small and tend to draw up into the wound, the surgeon probed for several minutes, but he found nothing else. Satisfied, he closed the wound with neat little stitches.

The wiring of the nervous system consists of microscopic hairs that sprout from nerve cells, like tails. A nerve cell can't reproduce itself, but it can grow a new tail.

The regrowth process is very slow—about an inch a month, the neurosurgeon told Josh's parents. Meanwhile, Josh would require some special care. Since he had no feeling in the arm and hand, he could easily cut, burn or frostbite it. He would have to wear a glove all the time, and his mother would have to examine Josh carefully each time he came in from playing. It would be an annoyance not only to Josh but to his family as well.

In a few weeks the sensation began to creep downward from the healing scar. The growing nerve tingled and itched. Sometimes it burned. Gradually the boy regained control of his arm and, finally, of his thumb and first two fingers.

But then, before sensation returned to the edge of the hand and the two little fingers, the improvement ceased.

For a while the local neurosurgeon was puzzled, but the truth soon became clear. The ulnar nerve must have been cut, too.

The surgeon wasn't sure what he should do next. A freshly severed nerve is relatively easy to repair, but once scar tissue has formed and degeneration begun . . . well, having failed once, he didn't feel competent to try it a more difficult second time. What was worse, he didn't know anyone else who could do it, either.

He confessed the problem to Josh's parents. They went home, talked about it, and refused to give up. The next day they started doctor-shopping. Many months and several surgeons later, a specialist in Philadelphia told them about Dr. Ducker.

Dr. Ducker, they learned, was chief of neurosurgery at the University of Maryland Hospital, in Baltimore. He had made a name for himself repairing peripheral nerves at Walter Reed Army Hospital during the Vietnam war. He later wrote the standard treatise on the subject.

A few weeks later the boy stood in Dr. Ducker's office, watching him carefully.

Baseball?

The neurosurgeon smiled and ran his thin fingers through his short, sand-colored hair. That sounded like a reasonable request. Of course, it wouldn't be easy.

No, sir.

The wound would have to be reopened, and Josh would have to wear a cast. It would hurt, and he would have to be brave.

Yes sir, said the boy.

And there was one other thing, too. Josh would have to understand that Tom Ducker had some college degrees, and that he considered himself to be a very good surgeon. But being a very good surgeon was not the same thing as being a perfect one. He couldn't promise miracles. Something might happen.

Yes sir. It might not work.

That's right.

But if it did . . . baseball?

Baseball . . . yes. Baseball was a reasonable goal to work toward.

Now Josh's name was on the operating room schedule. Number twelve. First thing.

In the grand old house in fashionable Guilford, Dr. Ducker turned over on his back and reviewed the diagnosis once again, more from habit than necessity. Removing ulnar nerves from scar tissue and restoring their function was an old, familiar routine. He liked the operation. He had worked out all his fallback positions, and he was good at it, the same way he was good with a sailboat. Tom Ducker always liked things he was good at.

He also liked things that were safe, and while something might always happen, the ulnar nerve was a long, long way from the brain stem. A long way from the soul.

Finally, reluctantly, he slid from beneath the covers. His feet searched briefly for his slippers. He closed the bathroom door before turning on the light.

As the sun rose, so did the Ducker household. Barbara was in the kitchen, doing something magical with a waffle iron, and his children's voices echoed down the halls. There was no smell of coffee. Tuesday was an operating day, and coffee made his hands shake. He showered, shaved, dressed, knotted a tie and removed a dark-blue jacket from its wooden hanger.

After breakfast he went out into the gray winter morning, carrying the brown paper bag that Barbara had wrapped his lunch in. It would be sailing season soon. Soon by the calendar, anyway. This morning there was a thin rind of sleet on the windshield, and spring was a fantasy. The station wagon started promptly, diesel smoke puffing from its exhaust. Its heater blew cold air.

The curving road wound between the old mansions of Guilford, then gave way to Maryland Avenue row houses. By the time the guard waved the station wagon into the hospital parking lot, it was warm.

Inside, he waited in the elevator corridor off the big main lobby. People nodded to him and he smiled back, absently, his mind on the coming operation. For a few minutes all the elevators seemed to be going down, toward the autopsy rooms in the subbasement. Then four upward-bound cars stopped at the same time and Dr. Ducker stepped into the nearest one. He got off on the seventh floor.

In the professors' dressing room he placed the paper bag on the top shelf of his locker and changed into a green scrub suit. A paper cap went on his head and booties went over his shoes. He picked up a face mask and pulled its rubber strap around his neck.

The nurse at the main desk nodded at him as he hit the pressure switch on the wall. The double doors swung open and he entered the surgical hallway.

He could smell the coffee in the nurses' lounge, but there was no temptation. Not only did the stuff make his hands shake, it made his kidneys work overtime. The public thought the brain surgeon needed good hands, and he did, but you'd wash out just as fast if you had flat feet or a weak bladder.

Dr. Ducker paused to peer through the window of Operating Room Eleven, next door to where he would be operating. A woman, already anesthetized, lay on the table. The senior resident was painting her shaved head with antiseptic. Dr. Michael Salcman, a dark-haired, square-jawed surgeon in his early thirties, was talking with Kay Donnelly, the circulating nurse, and Doris Schwabland, the scrub nurse.

Dr. Salcman was Dr. Ducker's second-in-command in the Division of Neurosurgery and Kay and Doris were the most experienced nurses on the staff. The neurosurgeons often argued over who would get those nurses on a given day, and the surgeon with the most complex operation usually won. Today it was only right that Michael have the first team.

The operating room personnel already had masks on, so Dr. Ducker pulled his own up over his nose before pushing through the door. He went directly to the X-ray board. In a few seconds, Dr. Salcman joined him.

The junior man had already scrubbed and gowned, so he remained well clear of Dr. Ducker. Except when pointing at the CAT scans he kept his arms crossed over his chest, his gloved hands tucked under his arms.

The tumor was a glioblastoma multiforme, a uniformly fatal brain cancer. The patient was forty-three, and had already had one operation to remove the tumor which, naturally, had reappeared. Today Dr. Salcman might buy her another six months, or even a year. But he wouldn't cure her.

The operation would be a continuously dangerous process involving an infinite string of decisions. The tumor was very near one of the areas that define personality, whatever that is. Michael, always the poet, called them "eloquent" areas. There was, as the word implies, a certain lofty beauty about such parts of the brain.

But it was the kind of beauty that was dangerous. He would have to remove each piece of tumor with extreme care, lest it be attached to something eloquent, something that shouldn't be disturbed. And he could never, under any circumstances, pull on anything.

The first rule of neurosurgery: Don't pull on anything.

It might, as Michael liked to put it, be attached to something. It might be attached to something that's attached to something that's attached to the soul.

As Dr. Salcman's team prepared to make the first incision, Dr. Ducker made his way through the autoclave room that connected the two neurosurgical suites. He was careful not to touch the hot front of the autoclave, where instruments were being sterilized.

Josh lay on the table, his eyes darting around the brightly lit room. Each time his heart pounded, one of the anesthesiologist's instruments emitted a clear beep. The beeps were coming very rapidly.

Dr. Ducker pulled the surgical mask down around his neck, walked over to the boy, and stood above him.

Fear is a chemical storm that rages through the brain, and a grin will sometimes still the waves. It is a thing a neurosurgeon learns as a resident, if not before.

Hesitantly, Josh smiled back. The heart rate slowed, very slightly.

"You already got an IV started, huh?" Dr. Ducker asked Josh, pointing at the needle in his right arm.

Josh nodded. The heart rate slowed more.

"Okay," Dr. Ducker continued. "You know how to count sheep or whatever it is you do?"

Josh nodded, solemnly.

"Sometimes," the neurosurgeon warned, "these particular sheep make your mouth taste funny. Don't worry if it does that."

The anesthesiologist pressed a plunger and Josh's eyes turned dull and rolled back, the lids closing. His head fell to one side.

The anesthesiologist moved quickly to insert a plastic tube into the boy's windpipe. Oxygen hissed through a valve. Dr. Ducker stepped aside to allow a male nurse to begin scrubbing the inside of the boy's arm with a foaming brown antiseptic.

Don't forget, Dr. Ducker told the team, to scrub the left leg as well. That way, if the two severed ends of the nerve were so atrophied that they wouldn't reach, he could take a piece of nerve from the leg, and put in a graft. That would leave the boy with a numb little toe, but that would be a minor loss. Josh could play first base with no little toe at all, if he had to.

Dr. Ducker went back outside to scrub. Standing in front of the big deepsink, he reached up and took a pre-soaped scrub pad from a dispenser. His knee automatically found the stainless-steel stirrup beneath the sink, slipped inside, and pressed to the right. Water splashed loudly into the porcelain basin.

The scrub is ritual. Ten minutes.

The neurosurgeon's eyes focused on the box of sponges in front of him, but his mind was far away, looking ahead, visualizing the scalpel and the cut it would make, remembering the scores of Vietnam soldiers at Walter Reed, reviewing once again the possible complications, the fallback positions, and always, always, the anatomy. The neurosurgeon who didn't know his anatomy perfectly was a menace.

Dr. Ducker remembered the patients at Walter Reed. Sometimes the neurosurgeon in the field hospital or emergency room hadn't properly reviewed the nerves of the arm and, in the excitement, spliced together the wrong nerve endings. The nerves regrew, but when the soldier tried to make a fist his biceps responded and the arm rose. When he tried to raise his arm, he made a fist instead.

Mistakes like that were easier to make than most people realized. The microscope magnifies the brain, revealing a new level of complexity, while allowing the surgeon's mind to focus down and get lost, if he wasn't careful, in the welter of detail. Fixated on a tiny, tiny problem, the surgeon can lose his bearings.

The experience is brutal, and few neurosurgeons escape it. Once, when he was much younger, Tom Ducker operated on the wrong side of a patient's spine. Fortunately it was an operation that did no damage to the nerve, so rectifying the error required no more than another operation. But such occurrences could be tragic. A luckless surgeon could become engrossed in the techniques of microscopic surgery and operate on the wrong patient.

At meetings and conventions, brain surgeons swap stories of neurosurgeons who got lost—who suddenly realized that the tumor they were removing wasn't, in fact, a tumor, but the brain stem itself.

It must be an awful, awful feeling, to hurt or even kill a patient with a navigation error.

Dr. Ducker scrubbed carefully and methodically. First he washed his hands, lathering with an abrasive sponge. Then, carefully, he rinsed.

Something . . . can always happen. Sometimes it's something unanticipated that begins with a little thing, and builds slowly, unnoticed, until the process has picked up speed and events come too rapidly to analyze, and you can't think fast enough. Then the thing that's happening, the whatever, the Something, is in control.

The neurosurgeon's foot pressed a rubber bulb on the floor and more soap squirted into his left hand. Now, using his clean hands, he washed his wrists and, in the process, re-washed the hands.

Sometimes, with no warning, something happens and there's blood in the field and Big Red, as they say, you meet Big Red, and instantly the OR gets very quiet and the staff tenses, waiting for orders from the surgeon. But there's little they can do to help when it's Big Red. You're alone.

Having scrubbed to mid-forearm, he rinsed again, carefully letting the water run away from his hands, toward the elbow, carrying the bacteria and the viruses all downward. Then he squirted more soap onto his hands, washing to his elbows this time.

Sometimes you didn't even know, after it's all over, what the something was. The operation went perfectly, the team worked together like a ballet troupe, and afterward you told the family the operation was a success, and then the patient died. Or had a sudden stroke, and couldn't move one side of his body.

All you knew was that something . . . something simple or something complex, something you worried about or something you didn't think to worry about, something odd or something you'd read about in dozens of articles, something . . . The brain has little in the way of an immune system, and is easily infected. Infection turns the brain to liquid.

Ten minutes. He didn't count them, he meditated on the operation to come, and when the scrub was over, he knew it intuitively.

Carefully, stepping back from the deepsink, Dr. Ducker raised his clean hands. Then, holding them in front of him, he backed through the operating room door.

The heart monitor beeped rapidly, regularly, steadily. It was a little too fast, but that often happened with children. Because Josh was a child, the anesthesiologist would keep him sleeping as lightly as possible.

The scrub nurse shook out a green wraparound gown and held it out for Dr. Ducker, who slipped into it and whirled, hands high, to wrap it around his body. The nurse tied it in back.

Most of the boy's body was already draped by green sheets. There was an extension fastened to the table, and the damaged arm was secured at a ninety-degree angle.

The resident sat on one side of the arm and Dr. Ducker sat on the other. The scrub nurse moved her tray of sterile instruments over the boy's hand, as close as she could get to where the incision would be made. The anesthesiologist sat amid his instruments on the other side of the table.

Dr. Ducker squirmed a moment on the stool until he felt comfortable, and reached for a scalpel. He held it lightly in his hand, surveying the arm.

There will be a great deal of scarring in the tissue beneath the wound, he told the resident. The detached ends of the nerve will be buried in the scar, and they won't be easy to find. The first few times you try it, he said, you won't see the nerve until it's pointed out to you. Even then you may have trouble seeing it. But you learn.

Dr. Ducker stared at the arm. With the tip of a gloved finger, he traced an invisible line along the soft flesh inside and above the elbow.

"Anesthesia okay?" he asked.

"Fine," replied the anesthesiologist, from amid his stack of monitoring equipment.

The clock on the operating room wall said 8:10.

Dr. Ducker's hand moved downward and the scalpel sliced cleanly through the skin, just below the scar. Blood welled up from the wound.

Dr. Ducker moved back, allowing the resident to search the wound with the tweezer-like electric cauterizer. Each time he caught a torn vessel—a bleeder—between the tips, the resident pushed a switch on the floor, and electric current arced through the blood vessel and welded it shut. The smell of burning flesh rose from the wound.

When the field was clear of blood the resident pulled open the wound and sat back. Dr. Ducker's scalpel sliced deeper.

The heartbeat was one hundred and ten, a little fast but rock-steady, normal for the circumstances, perfect.

A medical student appeared in the operating room and asked if he could watch. In a few minutes, he was joined by another.

As Dr. Ducker alternately deepened the wound and waited for the resident to tie off the bleeders, the neurosurgeon pointed out anatomical landmarks. The clock on the wall moved slowly. The surgeon's voice was calm and relaxed.

"Now take a nerve like the ulnar," he said. "It's a message trunk line far more complicated than anything Ma Bell ever dreamed of putting beneath the streets of New York. The individual circuits are carried by the axons, which are the tails that grow from peripheral nerve cells at either end of the trunk line. The electrical tails are so small that it takes an electron microscope to really get a good look at one.

"Most of the nerve, like most of the brain, is white matter. The white matter of the nerve is made of what's called Schwann cells."

Schwann cells are the servant class of the nervous system. They wrap the axons, insulate them, cushion them, even feed them.

A nerve like the ulnar is about as big as a piece of spaghetti. If you cut a nerve you can look at the ends of it and see several little bundles of axons traveling down through it in special channels.

"But the thing to remember is that it's a cable for transmitting messages. After you've seen the cut end of a nerve, you'll see what I mean. It even looks like a telephone cable."

In this case, the surgeon predicted, separating the ends from the scar tissue is going to be like removing a piece of overcooked spaghetti embedded in gristle.

The resident poked in the scar tissue.

"I don't see a thing," he said.

Dr. Ducker peered at the wound but he didn't see the nerve either.

"Scalpel," he said, holding out his hand. He would try well beneath the scar, and follow the nerve up the arm.

"When a nerve is cut," he explained, "the axons above the cut try to grow, but don't go anywhere. Sometimes when you reoperate on a patient like Josh, here, you find a knot of tangled axons right above the scar. They tried to grow down and make contact with the numb hand, but they couldn't get by the scar."

In the meantime, he continued, the axons below the cut atrophy and disappear. The white cells start to die out, too, but they're a hardier breed and the spaghetti-like nerve stays more or less intact for some time. It's like you took a message trunk line and pulled all the wires out of it, leaving holes surrounded by insulation.

A good neurosurgeon can cut out the scarred area, and match the raw ends of the nerves, and sew them together. If you do it right, the neurons will find the channels and grow down them at about an inch a month. They will eventually get down to the hand, and Josh will be able to play baseball.

Dr. Ducker handed the scalpel to the resident and took over the cauterizer.

Go ahead. Carefully.

The resident cut into the arm, carefully, each move watched by six pairs of eyes. As he worked, Dr. Ducker encouraged, warned, chided, and taught.

Gently, the neurosurgical chief said. Easily. Let it come to you. Don't pull on it, don't ever pull. Lift. Coax. Slide.

The heartbeat monitor beeped rapidly, one hundred and ten beeps a minute, steady, strong.

The resident bent over the wound, absorbed. Minutes passed.

Never taking his eyes from the resident's hands, Dr. Ducker encouraged him. Keep looking. You'll find it.

But it should be right there, the resident complained. It should be right there, right where the anatomy book said it should be.

But it wasn't.

Dr. Ducker commiserated.

Without warning, a high-pitched whine blasted through the autoclave room.

Zhooop . . . zhoop . . . zhoooooooooooooooooooo. Zhoop-zhoop. ZHOOOOOOOOOOOOOOOOOOOOOOOOOOOOOOOOOOOOOOO OOOOOOOO

The craniotome. In OR 11, Michael was opening the skull.

Zhoooooop, zhooooooooooo.

An air drill sounds very much like a tire shop impact wrench, and is discordant in a neurosurgical operating room. The circulating nurse closed the door. The resident remained bent over Josh's arm.

Zhoooooooooooooooooooooooooo. Zhooo. The door muffled the noise of the craniotome, but didn't stop it.

Keep at it, Dr. Ducker said to the resident. Keep at it, carefully, slowly.

Zhoooooooo. ZhoZhooZhooooZhoooooooooooooooo.

The ulnar looks enough like everything else that if you don't watch your anatomy, you can miss it and, with a single touch of the knife, slice through it. Then the odds on Josh playing baseball would go down, way down.

"I don't see it."

"You will. Cut right there."

Dr. Ducker settled down on his stool.

ZhoooooooooooooooooOOOOOOOOooooooooOOOOOOO. Zhoop.

Patience, said the chief of neurosurgery. Careful. Don't let yourself pull on anything. You never know what it might be attached to.

CHAPTER

THREE

If Tom Ducker had been able to work up any enthusiasm over writing and spelling, he might have followed his father and brother into the practice of law. Then he might have been arguing malpractice cases instead of bending over the arm of an eleven-year-old boy, patiently reminding a junior resident to be gentle, gentle, always gentle.

Don't pull.

Coax it.

Let it come to you.

Someday, in just a few more years, if he is gentle enough, and studies hard enough, and pleases Dr. Ducker enough . . . and if he's lucky enough, because something can always happen . . . if all those ifs are satisfied, then someday the resident will be a neurosurgeon.

It's not enough just to be smart and ambitious, of course. By the time the student gets to medical school everybody around him is smart and ambitious. In medical school, students are no longer weeded out, they are selected.

From the student's point of view, it is a process of professional self-discovery. One of the things he finds out is whether he's a talker, a cutter or a toucher. If he's a talker, psychiatry awaits him. If he's a toucher, he will choose internal medicine. If he's a cutter, of course, he will cut.

With the passage of time the doctor forgets many of the daily details of medical school, but he remembers the pivotal events with crystal clarity.

Tom Ducker, for instance, will never forget the dog.

It was sort of a mongrel collie, and Tom's sudden appearance into its previously drab life sent it into ecstatic, wriggling motion. It pranced on the tabletop, its tongue hanging out and its tail wagging. Its claws clattered noisily against the stainless-steel surface. Tom and the other medical students looked at one another, guiltily.

The curriculum decreed that the class would be divided into groups of three. One student would be the surgeon, the second would be the assistant, and the third would be the anesthesiologist. If the dog survived and recovered the students would rotate their responsibilities and do another procedure. In this fashion, the curriculum said, each student would do each job three times before the end of the year. For the dog, that was a total of nine operations.

The curriculum didn't say a damned thing about who would cut first.

Tentatively, Tom Ducker reached out and scratched his first patient behind the ears. Gratefully, it slobbered on his arm.

Tom Ducker took a deep breath. He knew his duty.

"I'll do it," he said.

And, he silently promised the dog, he'd do it well. That night he sat in his room, his anatomy and surgery books open in front of him. He would have to work quickly, he knew, but speed would have to be balanced with caution.

On the appointed day his scalpel cut cleanly through the abdomen. The assistant pulled the cavity open, revealing the glistening, moving, viscera. Tom pushed aside a loop of intestine and peered deeper into the cavity. The spleen was right where he thought it would be.

Carefully, but with a neophyte's awkwardness, Tom and the assistant tied off the blood vessels that fed the spleen and then cut it free. Tom sewed up the incision, placed a bandage on it, and the operation was finished. The next day the dog, weak and sore but healthy, licked his hand.

The first blood having been shed, the next student was not nearly so apprehensive. But he should have been, because after the operation the dog lay for days, consumed by fever, at the edge of death. The students had to sacrifice precious sleep to nurse the pitiful animal through the night. Every day the professor came around, looked at the dog, and lectured the students on what they were doing wrong.

Finally the dog was strong enough for the third operation, but again he suffered postoperative complications and the students had to resort to heroic measures to keep it alive. The dog became a terrible chore that had to be tended constantly. But they couldn't just let it die. Woe betide the medical students who let their dog die.

Finally, after a long recovery, the dog was strong enough for Tom to do his second operation. It went well. Afterward, the dog weakly wagged his tail. In a week it was almost healed.

The other students got together. Tom Ducker was appointed permanent surgeon, and what the professor didn't know didn't hurt him.

In fact, the fellow was pleased as the dog came through operation after operation with its tail still wagging gamely.

Of the three students one became a cardiologist, one became a neurologist, and one became, many grueling years later, a neurosurgeon.

The dog operation, like the cadaver that must be dissected, is at bottom a mechanism for sorting medical students. Neuroanatomy, the study of the architecture of the brain, is a test of a different sort.

The neuroanatomy course is, first and foremost, difficult. In the last twenty years, as scientists have used new tools to probe the function of the brain, detailed knowledge of what it is and how it works has increased by orders of magnitude. At least in broad form, the new knowledge must be pounded into the young minds of the next generation's doctors.

For most students neuroanatomy is another course to survive, by decree of the dean. But the brain is something more than a mere organ, and its magical qualities raise deep, philosophical questions—just the sort of questions to attract young and inquisitive minds. In every neuroanatomy class, a few hear a siren song.

But they don't hear it from Dr. Marshall Rennels. Absolutely not.

In that respect, neuroanatomy as it is taught today at the University of Maryland is no different from when Dr. Ducker was a student.

There have been superficial changes. Dr. Rennels' classroom is a bright new hall, with projectors that can flash an endless procession of slides onto a screen. Dr. Rennels himself, a tall fellow with a shock of gray-brown hair and a quick grin, looks more like an English professor than someone who makes his living by cutting up dead human brains.

At Maryland, neuroanatomy is scheduled for the second semester of the first year. The timing is ingenious.

Baltimore winters are gray and slushy, and January is almost exactly equidistant between last summer's vacation and next summer's vacation. By January the embryonic doctor is so totally immersed in the business of medical school that he may have forgotten why he enrolled. He's too old for fantasies and too young for wisdom, his self-esteem is at its low ebb, and his defenses are down. That's when Dr. Rennels gets him.

Most of the students arrive early for the first lecture. They shuffle in their seats, arranging their overcoats, gloves, scarves, knapsacks and books. As the second semester begins the class has settled down into a coherent tribal group, and there is considerable traffic in shared pencils and notes.

Nobody warns them about the siren.

As Dr. Rennels steps into the room the shuffling stops and the voices die down. Dr. Rennels taps on the microphone, and the speakers thump loudly. For a moment he lets his eyes wander across the auditorium.

In medical school, unlike in college, a class stays together from beginning to end. They form distinct, coherent social groups with individual mob personalities, and the professors quickly classify and analyze each one. Marshall Rennels knows, before he steps on the stage, whether this is a dull class or a bright one, a clinical one or a scientific one.

Likewise if there are troublemakers, Dr. Rennels has been forewarned. If someone needs special consideration or help, he's been made aware of it. If there is a genius in the class, his reputation has preceded him.

By the time he gets the class, Dr. Rennels knows a lot about it and the individuals who make it up. But he doesn't have the faintest idea who will hear the siren, and who will not.

Dr. Rennels stands on the stage, microphone in hand, surveying the more than one hundred upturned faces. He could warn them, but he doesn't. It wouldn't do any good.

Instead, he talks about big words.

Words like "arachnoid," "dura mater" and "pia mater," the three membranes that wrap and protect the brain. Collectively, they are called the "meninges." An infection of the meninges is, of course, "meningitis."

Words like "foramen," which simply means hole. Words like "cortex," for the convoluted folds of data-processing cells that cover many of the brain's structures. Words. Big words. Lots of them. The students scribble notes.

He tells them what his first anatomy professor told him almost a generation ago, that they are about to increase their vocabularies by five thousand words. The words are as necessary as place names to a mapmaker. The brain is a mere two-and-a-half-pound handful of gray and white goo. But when examined closely its substance is as complex and as interrelated as the ecology of planet earth.

It has been mapped by generations of anatomists, and, unfortunately for the medical student, many of the pioneers gave different names to the same place.

The internal cerebral veins, for instance, join to form the *vena cerebri magna,* or great cerebral vein, which is also known as the Vein of Galen. Broca's area, which you might also call the inferior frontal gyrus, makes the lips and tongue move to speak. Wernicke's area, or the superior temporal gyrus, translates the spoken word into the brain's internal computer language.

Periodically, neuroanatomists from all over the world meet to negotiate standard names for the anatomical structures in the brain. The delegates always agree to a simplified language, then go home and continue calling things exactly what they've always called them.

Dr. Rennels' students are fortunate, in that Dr. Rennels prefers the anglicized version of the Latin words. In his mind, a name like *fasciculus dorsolateralis* is pretty stuffy. He prefers the easy informality of "dorsolateral fasciculus," instead.

The intricate, detailed nature of the brain shapes the personalities of the scientists who study it. Such scientists are, it seems to the student, grotesquely perfectionist. For instance, early anatomists found that there was some sort of fluid in the spine, so they named it spinal fluid. But when later scientists found that the liquid was made and stored in the brain, they weren't content to stick with the old, simple "spinal fluid."

Since it was in the brain, or cerebrum, as well as the spine, the name just had to be changed to cerebrospinal fluid. In practice, that becomes CSF.

Laymen, of course, can call it spinal fluid and hang the professors and their nit-picking. The medical student doesn't have that luxury.

This is a tough course, Dr. Rennels cautions. Keep up with the class. Don't get behind, or the information will swamp you. Obediently, the students bend over their notebooks, writing.

Dr. Rennels is popular among the students, who consider him a humane and lucid lecturer, adept at the art of keeping students awake. He's tolerant of stupid questions (as long as they're not *too* stupid), willing to patiently explain a thing twice or three times, or however many times it takes to erase the blank stares before him. He does the best he can to make the information hang together, and if it really doesn't, the students don't fault Dr. Rennels for not trying.

The brain, they perceive early in the course, is a subject of infinite complexity. As life begins the fertilized egg develops into a fetus, the dividing cells form a hollow ball, which then creases and folds in on itself. The protected interior of the infolded surface eventually becomes the nervous system.

The first brain cells divide rapidly, and their progeny swim deeper into the hollow interior of the crease. As surely as salmon find their way to the spawning ground, the embryo nerve cells migrate to the correct place in the skull and then, at exactly the right moment, begin to reproduce.

The migrating gray neurons are followed by white glial cells, which are destined to serve them. But the glial cells multiply slowly, now, leaving the available nutrients to the aristocratic gray cells. For intelligent life, the first biologic priority must be the neuron.

While this is occurring in the fetal head, other cells are growing downward, forming a long tail that will in time be encased in vertebral bones and become the spinal cord.

The brain and its tail, Dr. Rennels explains, are called the central nervous system. The nerves of the rest of the body carry messages to and from the central nervous system, and make up the peripheral nervous system.

The students take notes feverishly. Four days a week they sit in the room and listen to Dr. Rennels.

As class follows class, Dr. Rennels shows an increasing number of slides. Most of them of slices of the human brain. He seems to have an endless supply of brain slices. And of big words.

Superior cerebellar peduncle?

Pssst . . . How do you spell that?

I can spell it. Do you know what it is?

It's the topmost bundle of nerve fibers that branches off the cerebellum. You know, the brachium conjunctivum. Remember?

Oh. Yeah. Of course.

For most of the students, neuroanatomy is one more mountain range to cross on the way to the promised land and a lucrative practice in gynecology or orthopedics. But for some, as they pore over their books late at night, the siren sings.

The questions, once asked, are compelling.

What is this protein computer, anyway, this two-pound lump of gray jelly that is aware of itself? What is the magic of the neuron, and what does that say about the human dilemma?

Those are Great Questions. For a bright young student in the sciences they are almost wondrous questions. They are mesmerizing, urgent, compelling . . . which makes it strange that an otherwise superior teacher like Dr. Rennels doesn't ever focus on that sort of thing. And neither do the books.

The student who becomes mesmerized learns the words quickly, as he reviews his notes in search of answers to the Great Questions. The brain is an organ, like any other, except for that almost spooky way all the neurons are tied together.

But it secretes thought. It secretes thought the way the kidneys secrete urine.

What is thought?

Who am I?

The answer beckons, just around the corner, a few dozen more big words away.

It has something to do with the neurons.

The neurons are simple enough, in their own way. Superficially they're similar to most of the other cells in the body. Like the other cells, they get their energy from tiny internal refineries called mitochondria. Neurons secrete things. Like all cells, they have specialized molecules on their surfaces for detecting hormones and other chemical messengers.

Those specialized molecules are called receptors.

Receptor. Now there's a word that will appear on a test.

Neurons are exquisitely sensitive to the touch of chemicals, and they work so hard at generating electricity and producing their own secretions that, untended, they can starve to death in minutes.

A kidney cell can live for an hour without oxygen, but a brain cell suffocates almost instantly. If its waste products weren't constantly removed by the white servant cells around it, it would poison itself. If the temperature rises or falls so much as a few degrees, the neuron dies. It has almost no ability to defend itself from viruses and bacteria and, beyond infancy, it even loses the ability to reproduce itself.

The most important living creature in the human universe is sterile. How ironic.

Use your imagination, Dr. Rennels urges. Make yourself small, much smaller than the point of a pin. Shrink yourself to the scale of the neuron.

It is not very impressive. At this scale the neuron is about the size of a football, and it's encrusted with what might be taken, at first glance, to be barnacles. It has a long, slimy tail that stretches off into the distance.

Professor Rennels says the barnacle things cover the cell, completely obscuring its outer membrane. They are not called barnacles, of course. Not barnacles. Boutons.

Bouton. Write it down.

Don't dare call them barnacles on a quiz.

But the barnacles . . . the boutons, boutons, boutons . . . can be pulled off very easily, because they're actually just floating above the surface. And beneath those boutons you find the surface membrane of the neuron.

Student ears prick up. Is that a trace of wonder and awe in the professor's voice?

The neuron's membrane is covered with receptors.

Receptors?

Those are the things, the little molecules, that make a cell sensitive to hormones and other substances.

All cells have them, of course. That's how they tell when to work hard and when they can loaf. Most cells have just a few.

But the neuron's membrane is covered with them? What does that mean?

The students write furiously in their notebooks. The implication is obvious: The neuron is exquisitely sensitive to outside influence from chemicals.

Why is it so sensitive? Where do the chemicals come from?

The thing to remember, Dr. Rennels says, is that if the neuron were the size of a football, then the skull cavity would be large enough to contain, oh, say, a half-dozen Astrodomes. And the neuron certainly isn't alone in there. There are billions, maybe trillions, of other neurons in there with it.

And they are all interconnected. The key is the tail—and the boutons.

The neuron's tail stretches off into the distance, perhaps to the other side of the skull, before breaking into many forks. Each fork has at the end of it a bouton, pressed up against the membrane of a fellow neuron. The tails are the wiring of the brain. The neuron synthesizes chemicals and pumps them down its tail for storage in the faraway boutons.

It also generates electricity. The charges fire down the tail, moving at very high speed, to jolt the boutons. Each time a bouton is jolted, tiny ports open on its underside. Powerful drugs flow out of these ports and wash against the sensitive membrane of the neuron beneath.

What are the chemicals?

Not chemicals.

Neurotransmitters. Another big word.

Neurotransmitters are messenger molecules. There are two basic kinds. One of them makes the cell work faster, and is a stimulant, like the caffeine in coffee or the amphetamine in diet pills. The other slows it down, and is called a depressant. Morphine is a depressant and so is Valium. Each cell makes only one kind.

But since the boutons that encrust its surface were put there by many different cells, the neurotransmitters that wash over the neuron's sensitive membrane are contradictory. Some stimulate it to go faster, others slow it down.

Dumbly, the cell averages the conflicting orders and behaves accordingly. If the depressant boutons are the most active, the neuron will work at a lazy idle, firing perhaps no more than one charge a second down its tail. If it's awash with stimulants it goes much faster, with a top panic speed of about sixty pulses a second.

Usually, though, the stimulants and depressants more or less cancel one another out and the neuron plods along at a moderate, consensus speed.

The tail of a neuron is an axon. Axon. Some tails . . . axons . . . are quite long, stretching all the way from the brain down to the tip of the spinal cord. Anything that small, and that long, is going to be very, very delicate.

Delicate isn't the word. There is no word to describe the delicacy of the brain cell, or of its tail. Touch it, and it tears and dies.

And there's no word that adequately describes the chemicals, either. "Neurotransmitter" is nice and long, and it sounds like it belongs in brain science, but it implies nothing of what those chemicals really are, and the impact they have.

Are long-distance runners really junkies? Do they stress their bodies to provoke the production of that wonderful, wonderful, good-feeling neurotransmitter morphine?

Neurotransmitters are love, hate, fear, anger . . . faith?

The pencil falters. The professor talks on, unheard.

There are perhaps a trillion neurons in the brain, each covered with thousands of boutons. Each cell is connected, either directly or indirectly, with all the other cells. A trillion cells, each sending a different frequency of signal down its tail, processing, massaging data . . . daydreaming.

". . . reticular formation."

What? What's that?

What did he just say about the reticular formation? Is that important?

Pay attention.

The reticular formation is a network of primitive neurons and nerve fibers in the brain stem, and it modulates the operation of the entire upper brain. It monitors signals coming in from the body, and sends them on to the correct processing unit higher up. It processes orders from the higher brain, simplifies them, and sends them off to the body. It controls breathing, heartbeat and digestion.

It puts you to sleep, and wakes you up.

The neuron is so sensitive and so specialized that it would never survive without the white glial cells. These members of the brain's working class come in all sizes and shapes, depending on their function. Some act as shock absorbers around the neurons, while others remove the biochemical garbage and prepare nourishment. One specialized glial cell flattens itself out like a pancake and wraps itself around the axon, again and again, providing electrical insulation.

It's the glial cells, Dr. Rennels says, that make up the white matter of the brain.

The lights go down, the slide projector clicks, and image after image of human brain slices appear on the screen. Each slice shows the complex arrangements of gray areas and white areas. The grays are predominantly neurons, and that's where the processing takes place.

The white sections represent the tangle of tails—axons—that compose the circuitry. As with electrical cables, there is more insulation than wire. In the case of the brain, the insulation, composed of glial cells, happens to be white.

Notice, Dr. Rennels coaxes the students, that the various twists and convolutions of the gray matter can be identified, and, of course, named.

The pointer rests on a dark area of a slice taken from high in the brain.

That's cortical gray.

The outermost convolutions of the brain are all gray. Different areas are responsible for different sorts of computations. Your eyes collect images but you "see" with the cortical gray at the back of your brain. That's called the "occipital region." A similarly unmarked area called the "motor strip" runs roughly in a band, from one ear over the top of the head to the other ear. The motor strip tells your muscles what to do, and if it's damaged, you're paralyzed.

As for the cortical gray in front of the brain, the prefrontal lobes, just behind and above your eyes . . . nobody knows exactly what that does, but if it's damaged there is a change in personality. You become listless, disinterested, and your personality subsides. You can live and work, but you can't woolgather, you can't love, you can't dream.

As the semester progresses the students who hear the siren approach Dr. Rennels, individually and in groups, and try to engage him in conversations about the Great Questions. He is polite, and chats for a minute, but his interests lie elsewhere.

He figures they will eventually give up. Finally, they do. But it's Marshall Rennels they give up on, not the Great Questions.

Venting their curiosity, the students drift together at campus beer halls. There, finally, they can use their new vocabularies to shed light on this fascinating business of axons and art, of Freud and Nixon, of brain stems and love, of cabbages and kings.

Hey, guys. Have you read about the thalamus yet? It regulates pain. Sometimes, when it's damaged by a stroke, or when a neurosurgeon touches it, the patient wakes up in agony.

It's not real pain, of course. It's all, as they say, in the head. But it's relentless and they scream, just the same.

Yeah, more beer. All around.

I grant you it's not a profound truth, and it doesn't say anything about the human condition, but isn't it *interesting?* I saw a patient like that the other day . . .

A patient?

. . . interesting and sad. Awful.

A patient! A real patient!

The junior medical student doesn't get to treat anybody, of course, but he goes on rounds, and he watches and listens. And somehow, when he stands by the bed of a young mother with damage to her reticular formation, the Great Questions about the soul seem immature. At the bedside, pain and death don't pose great questions, they present brutal truths.

As his education progresses, the student who is absorbed by the brain discovers the neurosurgical suites.

Such a student learns that he is welcome, if he touches nothing and says nothing, to stand behind a surgeon like Dr. Salcman, or Dr. Ducker, and watch. Some students, better fitted perhaps for neurology than neurosurgery, are repelled by the experience.

Others are mesmerized.

The medical student watches the surgeon whittle away at a tumor with the patience of a watchmaker, or clip off a deadly aneurysm with the boldness of a matador. He sees death and it shakes him, so when he sees success he is all the more impressed.

On a normal day, a neurosurgeon will save a life.

A life. A human life.

The medical student stands back, respectfully, as the neurosurgeon passes.

Listening much, saying little, he picks up the ethic of the neurosurgical operating room. To cut into the brain you have to be very intelligent, and very disciplined, and very, very cool. You have to be cool because, in neurosurgery, something can always happen.

Also, and by the way, a neurosurgeon rarely if ever talks about the soul. Let yourself woolgather for an instant and something will happen—Big Red, or you'll touch something that's attached to something and the monitors will go wild, but by that time it'll be too late.

Neurosurgeons don't discuss the soul. They leave that to priests and first-year medical students.

The student stands back, carefully keeps his mouth shut, and learns.

Before you operate, you have to stand in front of the sink and visualize the brain. You have to be able to turn it over in your head, see it from all angles, know all the relationships. *The neurosurgeon who cannot do this is a menace.*

For a long time the would-be neurosurgeon is acutely embarrassed about his preoccupation—his previous preoccupation, rather—with mushy, impractical, unscientific questions about the soul.

Never pull on anything. Ever.

It might be attached to something.

By the time the medical student has become a doctor, then a surgeon, then finally a resident, working under the patient eyes of Dr. Ducker, he has all but forgotten about the Great Questions. He is no longer even sheepish about his youthful innocence.

He was, after all, young. Very, very young. And it was a very human mistake, a very easy one to make.

There was a Great Truth, all right, but it wasn't very arcane. He learned it in the OR.

All the brains in Dr. Rennels' laboratory were embalmed. But in the operating room they glisten and pulse and bleed and die, and each one contains a frightened creature not unlike himself.

CHAPTER
FOUR

In Operating Room Twelve, Dr. Ducker settled himself comfortably on the stool, watching the resident. The resident remained bent over the eleven-year-old boy's arm, looking for the ulnar nerve below the cut, finding nothing.

Minutes passed. Dr. Ducker's eyes never wavered from the resident's hands. Patience, the senior neurosurgeon counseled, as the resident became increasingly frustrated. Patience.

Sure, the ulnar nerve looks exactly like everything else in there. But it hasn't had time to wither away, so it's there, and you'll find it.

The resident probed, forcing himself to go slowly, carefully. It would be easier if he could test things by pulling on them, but he didn't. Tugging on something would only get him a reprimand, and reprimands add up.

The resident's ears heard the muffled zhoop-zhoop-zhoooooooooooo-ooooooo of the craniotome, next door, but his mind didn't register the sound. For him, there was no operation going on next door. There was no next door, no world beyond the complex anatomy of Josh's arm and Dr. Ducker's watching eyes.

Suddenly, Dr. Ducker called a halt.

"Right there. See it? There it is."

The resident stared. "I don't see anything."

"That's it," Dr. Ducker reassured him, "I guarantee you. It's small because it's atrophied, but it's the ulnar nerve. I know it looks exactly like everything else in there, but that's it."

"I'm sorry," the resident stammered. "I still don't . . ."

Dr. Ducker pointed. The resident looked across the gloved fingertip. Instantly the expression on his face changed to surprise.

"Well . . . I'll be damned."

Of course. Once you saw it, it was so obvious!

You see, the senior surgeon said, it's much smaller than it should be. It wastes away, atrophies, when it's not connected. If it stays disconnected for a year or more, it degenerates so much you can't graft it back.

The resident nodded. Once he saw it . . . how could he have missed it?

It's easy, Dr. Ducker reassured him. The suburban neurosurgeon missed it, remember? And the wound was still fresh then, so he didn't even have to contend with scar tissue. And it was still full-sized.

Look at it very, very closely, so you'll never miss another one.

The nerve below the cut was exactly the same macaroni color of the scar tissue, but once the resident knew what to look for he could see it. It was encased inside a thin, tough sheath of membrane.

Carefully, with Dr. Ducker watching, the resident teased the scar tissue away from the sheath. Minutes passed, a half hour. The noise of the craniotome stopped, but he didn't notice.

Once the nerve was clear on both sides of the scar he used a tiny pair of scissors to cut through the sheath. Carefully he lifted . . . lifted . . . not pulled, not lifted, beckoned . . . and the long strand of nerve came free.

He worked downward, along the arm. Dr. Ducker held the bipolar tweezers and burned the occasional bleeder closed. The nerve extends down the inside of the arm and around the inside of the elbow. That's why the elbow has a sensitive "crazy bone."

It was slow, tedious work but finally the nerve was free all the way down to just below the elbow. Then the resident extended the incision upward, toward the boy's armpit, and separated out the healthy nerve above the cut. As the nerve came free, Dr. Ducker covered it with wet gauze, to keep it from drying out.

What they were going to do, the chief neurosurgeon lectured, was to cut away the scarred ends of the nerve. Then they would stitch the raw ends together.

That would make the nerve shorter, however. If that problem was ignored, the ulnar would tear apart again the first time Josh extended his arm to catch a baseball.

To compensate for the shortening of the nerve, they would reroute it around and through the muscle in the hollow of the elbow. That should gain about an inch of slack. It would also deprive the boy of a crazy bone in that elbow, but he probably wouldn't complain.

As he worked, the resident monitored his chief's words, but he'd heard them all before. He heard them at rounds, and again yesterday in the hallway, and again this morning, and several times since then. But the medical students listened attentively.

The running account of the operation was also directed at the operating room team. The Ducker approach to neurosurgery held that everyone in the OR should know exactly what was going on at all times.

That was one reason why the room next door, where the more serious operations usually took place, had a television monitor. The medical students and visiting doctors could, by watching the monitor, look right down the surgeon's microscope with him.

A nerve is very much like a telephone cable, the chief neurosurgeon explained. That's how you tell when you've trimmed off all the abnormal tissue on the scarred ends. In a normal nerve you can see those little channels in the white tissue, filled with gray axons. It looks just like a telephone cable.

In the case of this boy, the severed end of the nerve won't have any gray. There'll just be holes, where the axons used to be.

The dissection out of the way, Dr. Ducker examined the scarred nerve ends. It was difficult to tell nerve from scar, he told the crew, but it looked as though the white Schwann cells had grown extensions toward one another. The thing had actually tried to regrow.

In Dr. Ducker's view that was one of the nice things about working on the peripheral nerves, as opposed to the central nervous system. When something dies in the brain or spinal cord, it stays dead.

But out in the body, in the peripheral nervous system, Mother Nature is a little more friendly to the neurosurgeon. Nerve cells don't regrow, but they can rejuvenate their tails. If you cut the scarred nerve ends back to healthy tissue and stitch the raw ends together very, very carefully, then, with a little luck and a lot of time, the ends will grow together.

Still, even when working in the peripheral nervous system, the resident knew better than to pull on anything. He must be careful, careful.

And he must have knowledge.

Sensation begins with antennae, nerve cell antennae, out in the flesh. They send sensations up the nerves to the spinal cord for transmission to the brain. There, the impulses are compared to stored information in the memory banks. Neurotransmitters flash through the brain as contradictions are hashed out.

Then, in only an instant, the brain responds. Marching orders flash downward, and the muscles move. A hand slaps a mosquito. Eyeballs shift. A salesman reaches out to shake a hand.

The resident knows all that and more, and he knows the long, Latin names for everything. Sometimes he slips and uses one of them at a party, and the person he's chatting with gives him a strange look. The resident knows quite a lot and is, in the rare moments when he has time to think about it, quite proud.

But in the course of his residency, the young surgeon comes to understand how little he really knows. It's not possible to actually *understand* the central nervous system, or even the simpler peripheral nervous system.

There are many things the big words don't communicate, things that only thousands of hours in the operating room will reveal—things like how to recognize the ulnar nerve when it's buried in scar tissue.

Ultimately a neurosurgeon must be in sympathy with the nervous system; he must know it as a pilot knows the sky, or a sailor the sea.

The resident was learning, under Dr. Ducker's calm eyes, the sense of the body as a complex ecology, a thing you could develop instincts about. You could learn to sense danger. You could even admire the scenery.

In ecological terms, the brain was a delicate subsystem, the most complex and sensitive of all. In its complexity and ingenuity, it resembled a jungle.

In the nervous system alone there were an astonishing number of distinct beasties, each with its own mission in life. Neurons, for instance. Some neurons were football-shaped, others were round, still others looked like pyramids, and some even had huge antlers.

As for their interconnections, they were so complex that they could only be described in broad terms.

Nature's way was beautiful and ingenious. His experiences first in the dissection lab and later in the OR reinforced the resident's fundamental respect for God's ability to do detail work.

Occasionally Dr. Ducker pointed out something of interest to the medical students, but mostly the operating room was silent, except for the rhythmic beeping of the heart monitor. A little fast, only a little, nothing to worry about. Kids respond that way, sometimes.

The circulating nurse arrived with two sets of surgical eyeglasses, and Dr. Ducker and the resident straightened up so she could slip them over their ears. The glasses were microscopic bifocals, with jewelers' loupes set into the bottom part of each lens.

Now the nerve was large, more like a tiny white snake than a piece of spaghetti. Dr. Ducker urged the resident to study the end of the nerve. It was solid. The holes, the chief neurosurgeon explained, were clogged with scar tissue.

Dr. Ducker showed him how to cut the tip off of the nerve, using a sterile wooden tongue-depressor for a chopping block. Then the two of them examined the raw end. Still no holes. While Dr. Ducker watched, the resident cut off another piece of the nerve. Again they examined the raw end.

There we go.

See?

The medical students leaned over Dr. Ducker's shoulder, straining to see. It was an awkward stance, a balance of risk against benefit. If a medical student didn't lean over far enough, he couldn't see. If he leaned over too far he'd touch the surgeon's sterile shoulder, and then, and then . . . Dr. Ducker's patience didn't extend to carelessness.

Even without the loupes the nerve ends looked like cross sections of telephone cable. It was exactly like Dr. Ducker had said it would be. There were five gray wires running through the nerve.

Three sets of eyes watched the resident slice the tip off the other end of the ulnar, the atrophied end. When he got past the scar tissue, Dr. Ducker held the nerve up so the students could see.

Just like the other side, only there were no wires, just empty holes. The axons, cut off from their parent cells far above, had withered, died and been absorbed back into the tissue.

The lower part of the nerve was smaller in diameter than the upper part, and there were only three holes, not five. Two channels had collapsed as the nerve itself began to wither away.

Not "holes," of course.

Fascicles.

The fact that there were only three fascicles left meant there wouldn't be room for all the nerves to regrow, said Dr. Ducker. He studied the raw end, thoughtfully.

But enough would. Enough, he thought aloud, for baseball.

The surgeons worked for a while in silence. Then a medical student said, deferentially, that something was puzzling him.

Uh-huh?

How can you graft a five-channel cable onto a three-channel one? The holes won't match.

They don't have to, Dr. Ducker explained. It was enough, in his experience, to sew the nerve together by its outer membranes, without regard to the holes inside. The nerve fibers would find their own way.

Those that go down the wrong fascicle and connect improperly wouldn't cause problems, he said. Within rather strict limits, the nervous system could correct for wiring errors. The brain reprogrammed itself to compensate. That was the theory, anyway. Josh's hand wouldn't work right at first. He'd have to relearn how to use it.

The scrub nurse opened a package of tiny, almost microscopic needles. They sparkled beneath the strong lights.

The trick is to be delicate when sewing the ends together, the chief neurosurgeon said. If you don't do it right they become inflamed and die. When that happens, scar tissue grows in and fills up the holes before the axons can grow through. Then you're back where you started.

It isn't enough to be delicate, of course. The sutures have to be placed correctly, in exactly the right place, or the nerve ends will pull apart.

Dr. Ducker examined the raw ends of the nerves. As is typical of the nervous system, the tissue was soft, almost a gel. Only the outside membrane, called the epineurium, was strong enough to hold a stitch.

Not just any stitch, of course.

The needle had to be tiny and the stitches had to be placed just so. It required a clear eye and a steady hand.

It was the sort of thing that Tom Ducker had always been good at. Being good at it, he naturally practiced it. Practicing, he naturally got better at it and, getting better, he naturally earned a reputation.

When Dr. Ducker regrafted a nerve, the word got around. That was what drew the medical students.

Now, as the scrub nurse laid out the needles, the circulating nurse went through the autoclave room and into the other OR. The chief resident, who was scheduled to assist Dr. Salcman, had asked to be notified when Dr. Ducker reached this stage of the operation.

The circulating nurse held the door open for him, and he came through with gloved, bloody hands held tightly against the sterile fabric on his chest. Without a word the medical students moved aside, yielding the best viewing position.

Dr. Ducker acknowledged the chief resident without looking up. Carefully, holding the needle in a pair of small tweezers, he ran it through the epineurium of first one end and then the other.

Gently, he pulled the sutures, and the cut ends moved a millimeter closer to one another. He pulled again, peering through the loupes, concentrating.

The heart monitor beeped steadily. High on the wall the second hand of the clock moved around, and around again.

The chief neurosurgeon's eyes gazed into the loupes, unmoving, cold, as his fingers pulled, carefully, gently, urging, beckoning . . . The nerves touched. His gloved hands moved quickly, and the stitch was tied.

Then Dr. Ducker's eyes moved upward, to the resident's face. Now. You do it.

Hesitantly, the junior surgeon took the tweezers and needle. When Dr. Ducker did it, each stitch took a long time. The resident took even longer. His hands shook, slightly, under the pressure.

For a polite moment, Dr. Salcman's assistant watched the junior resident fumble with the needle. Then he glanced at the clock and, saying nothing, turned and went back to his own patient. Dr. Ducker's eyes didn't stray from the nerve, the needle, and the resident's hands.

That's right, he said. Good . . . Turn it over . . . Another stitch right there. No, there . . . Right . . . Gently, gently, gently.

The OR team worked smoothly. The clock inched forward and the heart monitor went beep, beep, beep, one hundred beats a minute, perfect.

No reason, Dr. Ducker mused, why this little fellow shouldn't be playing first base in, well, say . . .

The axons would grow at the rate of an inch a month, and they wouldn't finally reconnect to the fingers for about a year. After that, it would take a few months for Josh's brain to reprogram the signals and reco-ordinate everything.

. . . say, a year from this coming summer.

Dr. Ducker relaxed on his stool, watching the resident, feeling comfortable.

Most of the time, it was different. Tense. You couldn't relax for a moment. You didn't dare.

When you were doing something like tying off an aneurysm or an arteriovenous malformation, the Something was always there, waiting for a misstep. Even if you planned carefully, and operated perfectly, the Something still got you one time in five.

Got you. Got your patient.

But with patients like Josh the Something was far away. The worst that would happen was that Tom Ducker would fail and Josh wouldn't get to play baseball, after all. But he wouldn't die.

He wouldn't die. It was a nice thing to know.

The heartbeat continued, one hundred, steady. The dials on the monitors jumped rhythmically. The scrub nurse arranged and rearranged her tools.

Dr. Ducker sat on the stool and watched the resident, coaching him, encouraging him, occasionally chiding him. The stitches went in one at a time, until eighteen sutures bound the two raw ends of nerve together.

Then the withdrawal began. First the nerve was tucked into its new channel. Then each set of muscles and membranes had to be pulled together and stitched into place. Along the way, the vessels had to be returned to their normal positions.

They closed the incision in the skin with small, neat stitches. As they bandaged the wound a nurse wheeled in a cast tray.

The cast would extend from the hand to the shoulder, Dr. Ducker explained to no one in particular. The arm would be bent, so as to minimize the strain on the fragile stitches. The resident applied the cast and an OR nurse wheeled in a bed.

Dr. Ducker held the arm for several minutes while the plaster warmed and set. When the cast was hard, the anesthesiologist stopped the flow of anesthetic and administered an antidote.

"Josh? Joshua?" Dr. Ducker called.

Josh lay still.

"Hey, Josh?"

The boy stirred slightly, and whimpered.

Carefully, Dr. Ducker lifted him from the operating table and laid him gently on the bed.

CHAPTER
FIVE

JOHNS HOPKINS CASE NO. 191-00-18 SAT ON THE EDGE OF HIS BED, ALONE in the ancient, high-ceilinged hospital room. He couldn't read, because the tumor pressed against the nerves that made his eyes focus. He couldn't walk around because the thing had loused up his co-ordination, and the nurses got hysterical when he bumped into things. They treated him like a baby, or some sort of delicate jewel, or a time bomb.

Well, they couldn't stop Joe Trott from thinking.

Six days, now. Six days of being poked and prodded, six days of sitting in wheelchairs and taking orders, of being zapped and scrutinized, six days, basically, of wasted time. He could have been finishing the spring quarter at Georgia Tech.

On the other hand, he couldn't have read an examination sheet. Even if he could have read it by closing one eye, he couldn't have made his hand write the answers. Not legibly, anyway. And even if he could have completed the exam it would have been tricky, trying to maneuver to the front of the room to turn it in. Somebody would have inquired, and then he would have had to see a doctor, and then the doctor would have called his parents.

No, it all came down to one thing. He had put it off as long as he could. There was nothing left to do but get it fixed, get it over with, and get back to school.

In the meantime, six days of boredom. They would be very solicitous if he couldn't sleep, and if he hurt, he was sure they'd give him some morphine or something. But boredom?

Didn't they know boredom was pain, too?

As he waited in the wheelchair, bored, he sometimes wondered— what was that thing growing in his head?

It didn't look like it was cancerous, Dr. Murray said. It was more like a soft wart, and it'd probably been there for years, since childhood perhaps. Perhaps it had been there when he was a fetus, a tiny patch of cells programmed to lie dormant for years and then, abruptly, to begin to divide.

The doctors had asked him about the timing of the first symptoms, but he honestly didn't know. The alien growth had made itself apparent so gradually that it didn't seem alien at all. But there were strange occurrences.

There was that time during his freshman year, for instance, that he lost his rat hat. The loss was surprising, even at the time. Joe wasn't accustomed to losing things, especially not things that were important.

The hat was a beanie made of gold cloth. Every serious freshman at Georgia Tech had to wear one, as part of the initiation process. The beanie identified you as a freshman, which was to say a rat, so it was called a rat hat. It was never called a beanie. That wouldn't have been cool.

Joe had heard of graduates who had had their rat hats preserved in bronze.

Joe liked the idea. Maybe someday he'd do something like that, one day when he was the vice-president of some corporation, or a wealthy entrepreneur. The rat hat represented a tradition, so it was definitely important, too important to lose.

Another grand old Georgia Tech tradition was the annual grudge football game with the University of Georgia. If you were serious about being a Georgia Tech freshman, you definitely went to that game and you definitely wore your rat hat. If you didn't understand that, you probably didn't belong at Georgia Tech.

The Grant Field stadium in Atlanta opens to the north, and that was the direction the icy wind was blowing that day. In deference to the weather, Joe put a stocking cap on his head and set the rat hat firmly on top of that.

The memory made him smile. It was a grand game, anyway. There were fifty thousand people in the stadium, and he saw many other rats. The afternoon sunshine glinted off the players' helmets, and illuminated their frosty breath as they lined up on the field.

In the stands, students and alumni alike jumped and waved pennants, screaming encouragement to the team and roaring with every Yellowjacket touchdown. Joe Trott leaped and screamed with them.

At eighteen, he was where he belonged and he knew it. He belonged in the stadium, watching Georgia Tech massacre its archrival. He belonged in the rat hat.

It was a great game, but as he left the stadium and reached up to remove his rat hat, it wasn't there.

Of course, there were explanations for his absentmindedness. Those were confusing times, because while he definitely fit at Georgia Tech he didn't necessarily fit as an engineer.

As a National Merit scholar, he'd chosen Georgia Tech as a good place to study engineering. Engineers built bridges, roads, sewer systems—they did practical things on a large scale, and weren't bothered by the ordinary pettiness of life. They seemed very strong, very much in control, very, well, cool. Joe thought he would fit right in.

But it wasn't turning out that way. The math seemed too theoretical, and he couldn't get interested. So maybe he wouldn't be an engineer . . .

But the Mr. Cool, hijinks attitude of the engineering student still suited him perfectly. He loved practical jokes—especially practical jokes that involved firecrackers.

Joe grew up in Maryland, where fireworks were banned, but in Georgia they're sold year round. To be a rat in a dormitory at Georgia Tech was to become intimately familiar with the stench of firecrackers. In this as in so many other things, Joe belonged. His creative mind weighed the possibilities, and was captivated. He understood intuitively that, while it was cool to explode firecrackers in the dorm, it was not cool to get caught.

Soooooooo . . .

It was cool, if you were Joe Trott, to be the Merit scholar, the quiet, studious fellow who, in the dead of night . . .

At two in the morning, when all is quiet, a firecracker makes a satisfying echo in the hallway.

Mmmff. I was asleep. Did something happen?

No, I didn't see a soul. Maybe they went the other way.

Who, me?

Only his closest friends knew that very little happened in the dormitory that Joe didn't know about. When something happened that was really ingenious, his friends assumed he was probably, at one level or another, involved.

His friends knew he was no milquetoast. They had to know. They played Dungeons and Dragons with him, and they saw the cold, Machiavellian fire in his eyes.

Dungeons and Dragons, in fact, was even more important to Joe than firecrackers. D&D is a creative and complex game based on imaginary characters who must be invented by the players. The characters are carried over from game to game, accruing attributes along the way. If the player is very good, his D&D character can assume bigger-than-life proportions.

Joe invented Anmar.

As he was guided through game after game, Anmar deepened and seemed to grow wise. With each crisis, he matured. With each dragon slain Anmar gained insight, until finally he developed into a powerful blend of wizard and philosopher-king.

Joe spent many hours with Anmar. Sometimes a game would stretch over an entire weekend. Other times Joe would lie alone on his bed, stare at the ceiling and devise new ways to make Anmar even stronger.

When he learned to use the campus computer he discovered a file, called "Forum," which was the cybernetic equivalent of a bulletin board. If you wanted a blind date, or had books to sell, you left the specifics in Forum.

Soon, strange messages appeared there. They were signed "Anmar."

Now *that* was cool.

If you learned nothing else of value in Georgia Tech, you learned the utility of being cool.

That didn't mean you didn't work, of course. Being cool was a lot more than firecrackers, football games and Anmar. Being cool was being a National Merit scholar, pulling eighteen credit hours, scoping out the professor.

It was also cool, Joe discovered, to climb down in a cave, to squirm through mazes of narrow passageways far underground.

With a group of spelunkers, he explored the netherworld of the earth, down where the bugs had no eyes and bats lived among the stalactites. Sometimes his fingers felt the floor drop away, and he tossed a pebble into the darkness and it fell, and fell, and fell, until there was a tiny, distant splash.

Some things, however, were uncool.

It was uncool to try to study your notes and find the penmanship so poor that it was undecipherable.

It was uncool to be sick.

You didn't get to be a National Merit scholar by going to bed and whining about every little thing. Besides, as he once told his mother, a cold or the flu is something you can put your mental foot down on.

Illness is something you can think away, if you have the power.

But that didn't seem to work on his deafness.

That came as a shock.

For some reason, without thinking why, he had developed the habit of holding the telephone to his left ear. One day, while taking a telephone message, he switched ears to free his left hand.

The caller's voice seemed unusually loud.

He shifted the telephone back and forth. There was no mistaking it. He heard better in his right ear than in his left. Now that he thought about it, in fact, he'd been straining to hear lately, cocking his head to make the best use of his good right ear.

The realization washed through his brain like ice water.

He was going deaf.

No.

Nonsense.

He didn't have time to go deaf.

It was probably wax in his ears.

That's what the doctor at the infirmary told him, the next day. He told Joe to rinse it out with hot water, and sent him on his way.

The hot water didn't help but, anyway, it apparently wasn't anything to worry about. A doc had examined him, and he didn't seem upset. Besides, there were classes, and caves, and firecrackers, and Anmar.

You couldn't be a scholar and the firecracker king of Georgia Tech if you spent too much time worrying about little stuff.

A trash can shapes the sound of an exploding firecracker, funnels it out into the room, bounces it off the ceiling. You can't ignore the solid KA-*THUMP* of a firecracker in a trash can.

One day Joe stood at the window of the dorm, staring vacantly at the ground, four stories below, his mind far away. For want of anything better, his eyes focused on a cigarette butt on the sidewalk.

Cigarette butt?

Two cigarette butts.

Or is it one?

Lazily, retrieving his attention from the land of Anmar, he idly examined the butt. Or butts. There seemed to be two, but not side by side. They were exactly alike, and they were overlapping. It was like two images of one cigarette butt.

He took off his glasses, rubbed his eyes, and put the glasses back on. Then he looked again. Now there was only one cigarette butt. Perfectly normal. Not something to worry about.

Neither was the deafness. It didn't respond to the power of positive thought, so he just didn't think about it. He could hear adequately out of one ear.

Joe discovered computer languages, first learning Fortran and later Pascal. Anmar survived another dragon, and another. With his friends, Joe explored Case's cave and Johnson's Creek cave, both across the state line in Tennessee. Spring finals came.

Exams were difficult, when you couldn't read your notes. But Joe Trott was a Merit scholar, and he made it.

Summer passed.

He thought a lot, and made some decisions. Industrial management, he decided, was much more appealing than engineering, and more practical as well. When autumn came and he was back at Georgia Tech, he changed his major.

After the confusion of his freshman year, the future looked bright.

But the present, by autumn, had become seriously compromised by his growing deafness. To compensate, he became more sophisticated at cocking his head and using his right ear to best advantage.

He found he could ignore the tiny insect that sometimes buzzed in his left one. He didn't try to get it out. He could tell, somehow, that it wasn't there.

As his symptoms got worse, he became haunted by the thought that he might be found out. If they found out, they'd take him out of school.

In his junior year, as his speech began to slur, he forced himself to talk more slowly. As his gait stiffened, he learned to avoid situations in which he might be expected to run. His double vision recurred, with increasing frequency.

Fortunately, it seemed to be isolated to the lower left quadrant of his visual field. Also, it only occurred when he looked at distant objects. Books, firecrackers and computer screens were plenty close enough to see.

As the symptoms got worse, Joe got better at concealment, but it became increasingly difficult not to think about them. Vaguely, he recognized that sometime, sometime soon, he would have to set aside some time to think through what was happening to him. Maybe even see a doctor.

Somehow, telling his parents about it didn't seem like a very good idea. They would probably overreact, and demand that something be done instantly.

Dropping out of school to be sick wouldn't be cool at all. He would have to go to a doctor and get it fixed, sometime when it was convenient. It certainly wasn't convenient now. Perhaps during his next school vacation . . . that way, he wouldn't miss any classes.

In the meantime the spelunking club put a notice on the bulletin board announcing an upcoming trip. Joe read the announcement once, then twice. He would like to go, but . . . would it be fair? In an emergency the others might need to depend on him and he would be too deaf, or too spastic, or too cross-eyed . . .

Damn.

The whole thing was beginning to annoy him. He would have to get it fixed, whatever it was. But not in the middle of the quarter.

He worried, though, about Christmas vacation. He would have to go home. His parents would demand it. And they'd pay a lot of attention to him. He would have to be careful.

His practice at looking innocent helped. He conspired to spend most of the vacation in his room, supposedly reading. Actually, he invested much of his time in thinking, fantasizing, listening to music, working out Dungeons and Dragons strategies and toying with his hand-held calculator.

His parents remarked about the change in their son. No practical jokes. No running around the house. Just studying, or quietly reading.

Perhaps Joe was maturing.

But it was a close squeak. By the time Joe arrived back in Atlanta, he was having trouble dressing. Finally, one morning, as he attempted to put on his trousers, he toppled over onto his bed.

Lying there, he finally looked at it squarely. Something was happening to his brain. Something serious. Chances were there was something growing in there, and that somebody would have to take it out somehow, and that was probably going to interfere with college.

No. They could do it during the spring break. He'd make some excuse to his folks, get it done then, get it done and over with, get back to school without missing a beat. He'd have to think of some phony reason why he wanted to stay in Atlanta. That shouldn't be difficult.

He called the infirmary for an appointment. No, there was no hurry. Early March would be best, actually. That would be two weeks before the semester break. March 3? Fine. Thank you.

It was difficult to keep the words from slurring.

March 3. That was good timing. That way they could get the tests over with and get on with the thing when the spring break began. Matter-of-factly, he organized a list of symptoms for the doctor.

It was difficult to read, to talk, to write, to walk. He tried to stay near railings and supports, so he could catch himself if he began to fall. More than once, his prudence paid off.

He began to look forward to getting it over with.

On March 3 he went to the clinic. When his name was called, he sat down in front of the doctor and told him that the deafness apparently hadn't been wax after all.

There was also the buzzing, and the balance problem, and his handwriting had gotten unreadable, and the double vision . . .

The doctor interrupted him. Double vision?

A little. Just a bit. And only in the lower left field.

But the doctor wasn't listening. He was rummaging through a drawer and assembling a hand-held instrument of some sort, with a light in it.

Look at the wall, please.

Joe did what he was told, and he sat there patiently while the man peered through the instrument and into his eyeball.

Presumably, he was examining the retina. Joe realized, uncomfortably, that the doctor's mood had changed. Joe knew the symptoms. The guy was . . . interested. He had been afraid of that.

In a few minutes, the doctor called in a colleague, and then another, to look into Joe's eyes. Joe obediently stared at the wall.

The infirmary doctors sent him across town to see a neurologist, some fellow who wore a big safety pin in the lapel of his white coat. At least the neurologist wasn't quite as fascinated as the infirmary docs.

Joe had the impression that this wasn't the first time this doctor had seen whatever it was that Joe had. He sent him right over to a local hospital, for a CAT scan. Afterward, Joe came back and sat in the waiting room until the scans were developed and delivered. By the time the nurse ushered Joe back into the office, the scans were hanging on the X-ray lightboard.

Joe sat down, his eyes on the images.

The tumor was fuzzy white, and while Joe could identify it easily, it looked small to him.

No, the neurologist said.

No. Not at all.

"Giant," was the word he used, followed by "acoustic tumor."

Joe moved uncomfortably in his chair.

"I guess," he finally said, "obviously, we've got to get this taken care of."

The neurologist agreed. He watched his patient think.

"Well," Joe said. "Can it wait until the end of the quarter?"

No, it couldn't.

Joe gave the doctor his parents' telephone number and watched him dial it.

March 3.

There was something about that date.

Oh. Oh, no. His mother's birthday.

"I am Dr. Lee," the neurologist said into the telephone, "and I am a neurologist in Atlanta . . ."

After a while, the doctor handed the telephone to Joe.

Mom?

Mom, I'm sorry. What a miserable birthday present for you. Joe's eyes rested on the CAT-scan images. It seemed like such a small thing, nestled in the bottom of the skull.

After the phone call, it was beyond Joe's control. His father drove down from Baltimore, which gave Joe just enough time to check out of the university. Then his father was making all the decisions, his father and other people. Joe, having no choice, did what he was told.

Two days after he went to the infirmary, he was in the Hopkins. Six endless, ignoble, boring days later, he sat on the edge of a hospital bed, thinking.

This is it.

Tomorrow I'm going to have brain surgery. They're going to mess with my head, take something out. If I'm going to get nervous, now is the time to do it.

Pause.

Well?

Pause.

If I go berserk and run screaming down the hallway, they're just going to grab me and sedate me until morning, and it won't make any difference.

Outside, a nurse pushed a rubber-wheeled cart quietly down the hallway.

Besides, it wouldn't be cool.

Joe Trott went to bed and slept soundly.

CHAPTER
SIX

THE CLINIC HAD QUIETED DOWN ABOUT 6 P.M. NOW THE ONLY SOUND coming through the counseling office doorway was the distant hum of a floor polisher. That's one of the things Richard liked about a night job. It gave him time to study.

He sat in a hard plastic chair, his head propped on his hand, eyes on the textbook. The coffee in front of him was cold, and the cigarette in the ashtray had burned down to a long, delicate ash. His gaze moved slowly down the column.

It was hard going, but interesting at the same time. And study was the only way he would ever be able to make something of himself.

The intercom buzzer startled him, and he hesitated a second before reaching over and flipping the switch. His other hand found a ball-point pen.

The chief nurse's authoritarian voice sent pulses of resentment through him, but he suppressed them. As he listened to her orders, he marked his place with an envelope, closed the textbook, and slipped it in the top drawer of his desk.

I'll be right there, he said when the nurse had finished. The intercom emitted a burst of static, and was quiet. Richard found an empty clipboard and placed a four-carbon admitting form in it.

There were two doors leading from the office, the open one that led out into the lobby and the closed one that led to the security area. He turned the knob and went through the security area door. It closed automatically behind him. On this side, there was no knob.

He padded down the silent hallway. At the end of the hallway, automatic doors opened in front of him and he walked through them into the lobby. The lobby had been designed before the energy crisis, and it was cold. The snowy March wind blew in beneath the door, and cold air wafted down from the plate-glass windows.

Richard shivered. He yearned for a hot shower.

The nurse stood bent over the admitting counter, writing something on a form. A middle-aged man in rumpled clothing stood in front of the counter, his hands behind his back. The fat policeman stood behind him, looking bored.

Richard's eyes scanned the patient, gathering information. The man stared tiredly at the nurse. His coat was threadbare, and he looked . . . unclean. Not dirty so much as unclean. As Richard moved toward him, the patient turned his attention toward the counselor.

Richard smiled. There was no smile in return.

Richard saw the cop reach for his handcuff key. Quickly, he spoke up.

"Remove the handcuffs, please."

The cop, the key already in his hands, hesitated. A momentary look of confusion crossed his face, and was replaced by a scowl. Reluctantly, he reached for the handcuffs. They made a metallic clicking noise as they sprung open.

Richard didn't mind the cop being irritated. He wanted the patient to think that he, Richard, was responsible for his freedom.

The man looked at Richard and rubbed his wrists. "Thank you, sir," he said.

Sir, huh? The patient called him sir. Very well. He would sir him right back.

The nurse handed Richard a folder, and he clipped it on the clipboard. Then he took the patient's arm, gently. We'll get this all straightened out, sir.

Richard guided the man through the automatic doors. The doors hissed behind them and closed with a sharp click. Down the hallway, the counselor used a key to open the door into his office.

Right this way sir, over here. Have a seat here by my desk.

The man did as he was told, but he didn't allow himself to relax. He sat stiffly on the edge of the chair while Richard took the folder from the clipboard and opened it.

It contained a copy of the police report, the emergency commitment papers and the nurse's orders. Richard placed the clipboard in front of him and began writing on the admission form.

Sir, the man interrupted. Sir, my rights have been violated.

Yes, said Richard, continuing to write. Cops do that sometimes.

The counselor glanced through the police report. The man was charged with making a public disturbance, which was police code for acting weird and getting in the way.

Just acting weird wasn't enough to get you hauled into the community psychiatric clinic. It was a lot of trouble for a cop to think up some nonsense charge, fill out the paperwork, explain everything to the judge, and get the commitment papers.

So you didn't get brought to Richard unless you were getting in the way. You had to be panhandling the mayor, or having fits in the middle of a shopping center, or . . .

Sir, my religious freedom is being infringed on.

I bet it is, Richard commiserated, his mind digesting the police report. Do you know the date?

The man stared at Richard.

He had been minding his own business, he complained, ignoring Richard's question. He had been preaching the word of the Lord Jesus God, and for that they handcuffed his wrists behind his back, locked him in a paddy wagon—

Richard interrupted. He leaned toward the patient, conspiratorially. He too, he confided, believes in the Lord Jesus God. And you know what? While Richard has never personally had the privilege, he has heard that some people can actually talk to God.

The patient stared at the counselor. For the first time, a glimmer of enthusiasm burned in his eyes.

God talks to me, he whispered, proudly.

Suddenly his voice rose an octave.

"Alas! Alas! Thou great city, thou mighty city Babylon! In one hour has thy judgement come."

I see, said Richard.

"And I saw a beast rising out of the sea with ten horns and seven heads, with ten diadems upon his horns and a blasphemous name upon its heads. And the beast that I saw was like a leopard, its feet were . . ."

Richard had heard theories that Christ had been a schizophrenic, but he doubted it. Sometimes, Richard reflected, the psychiatrists made sense, and other times they were full of shit. There was no resemblance, no resemblance at all, between Christ and the man now sitting beside him.

". . . its feet were like a bear's and its mouth was like a lion's mouth, and to it the dragon gave his power . . ."

Richard shifted his attention to what he was getting paid for, which was filling out the triplicate form. The patient seemed happy enough, reciting the Bible. The old fellow was no trouble at all.

As the man recited Revelation, Richard transferred information from the police report onto the health department admissions form.

The questions he couldn't answer he left blank. Later, when the man came out of seclusion, Richard would have to ask him where he'd been treated previously.

He had definitely been treated somewhere before. Of that, there was little doubt. Schizophrenics rarely had their first attack this late in life. Usually the brain disease struck in the teenage years, or the twenties, and it got better and relapsed, got better and relapsed, over and over, in and out of hospitals.

This fellow had probably stopped taking his Thorazine, which was why he was talking to God. Or, perhaps, he quit taking his Thorazine because he felt he needed to talk to God again. Richard wouldn't mind talking to God himself, some Mondays.

Richard stopped writing.

There was an irony in this, an irony in having a former drug addict treating schizophrenics. Some folks, like Richard, got into trouble because they took drugs to alter their minds. Others, like the preacher here, fouled up when they didn't. But it was only natural that they understood each other.

Several years ago, as he was learning to live without heroin, Richard had been fascinated by a description of brain chemistry in a popular magazine. The article said the mind functioned by squirting chemicals at its various parts.

Neurotransmitters, the scientists called them. In Richard's world the words were briefer. Heroin. Speed. Acid.

The preacher here, for instance, was a speed freak. Speed was amphetamine, an "upper," the stuff they put in diet pills, and Richard had seen guys hooked on it. They heard voices, and talked to God, and saw things, and had revelations.

The main difference between them and the preacher was that the preacher didn't buy his dope. He manufactured his own. In his head. It was no different than manufacturing too much growth hormone, or too little insulin. It was probably genetic.

When Richard began his psychological training in earnest, he was interested to note that the scientific breakthrough behind all that happened right in his own home town, Baltimore. It had happened over at Johns Hopkins.

The scientists had been Dr. Solomon Snyder and Dr. Candace Pert. Richard had read about them in the newspaper and in several magazines, as well as in his texts. He had become so interested at one point that he'd actually gone to the library and read the original scientific paper himself.

The paper was hard going, because instead of the familiar language of psychiatry, it was written in chemical terms. He had cursed that fact as he tried to puzzle out the meanings, but at the same time he had appreciated its significance. Imagine, psychiatry in the language of chemistry!

One day, treating the mind might be a hard science.

". . . and one of the four living creatures gave the seven angels seven golden bowls full of the wrath of God . . ."

Doctors Snyder and Pert hadn't discovered the existence of neuro-chemicals, exactly. Those had been postulated for years. What the Hopkins group did was demonstrate how they worked in the brain. The key was receptors. The Snyder-Pert team had learned how to label them chemically, and define how they worked.

The receptors were little molecules on the surface of the brain cells, and each one was sensitive to a certain chemical. That one chemical, and no other, would fit into the receptor like a key. When that happened the cell would be stimulated, or depressed—depending on the chemical.

The first receptor they'd found was for the natural form of morphine. A few months later, some researchers in England had identified the natural morphine itself.

There were a lot of other receptors discovered later, of course, and many more neurotransmitters. The interesting thing was that different cells had varying numbers of receptors for different functions. The emotional system, for instance, was rich with receptors for morphine and its analogs, like heroin. The brain stem, which regulated the rest of the brain, was very sensitive to something called dopamine.

Dopamine was probably what the preacher's brain was making too much of. The difference between dopamine and speed was not worth discussing.

Richard read somewhere that what Snyder and Pert did was going to change the world. That, Richard doubted. The world, in Richard's view, never really changed a whit.

"How long, O Lord," pleaded the preacher, "O Lord, holy and true, dost Thou not judge and avenge our blood on them . . ."

Richard studied him for a moment, and made a decision.

How, he asked, did they violate your rights?

The man stopped in mid-verse.

Tell me how it happened. Maybe I can help. I'll help if I can.

In a few minutes Richard had the man talking angrily about the way he had been treated by the cop. As he listened, the counselor correlated what the preacher said with what he read in the police report. Apparently, factoring out the conversations with God and translating the cop jargon in the police report, the preacher's conversations with God had been going on for several days.

He'd started off preaching on street corners in South Baltimore. As the hallucinations became increasingly florid, he'd moved downtown, attracted by the crowds, the neon, and the occasional coin a passerby would press into his hand. Sometimes he'd preached in front of topless bars. He ate in soup kitchens and hurt nobody.

The preacher's mission had come to a sudden halt, however, when the spirit called him to preach to the well-dressed couples patronizing a fancy new French restaurant.

Richard knew the place, though he had never been able to afford to take his wife there. Someday he would, after the baby was born. It was supposed to be very nice.

But the preacher was definitely out of place. Presently the maître d'hôtel emerged and ordered him to be gone.

The schizophrenic quoted a few verses at the maître d', then turned to buttonhole two more customers.

The maître d' pushed the schizophrenic aside and ushered the customers through the door. Inside, he picked up the telephone and called police headquarters. Presently the cop, who had been directing traffic a half a block away, arrived to investigate the situation.

Move along, the policeman told the preacher.

The preacher asked the cop if he had been saved.

The cop turned to the maître d', shrugging. He couldn't arrest the man for preaching. Preaching was legal.

You can't arrest someone for praying in public, unless . . . the maître d' might want to come down to central district and swear out a warrant, and then, at some point, when there was time, central would send somebody out with the paddy wagon.

The maître d' hesitated. That would take hours. The tips he would lose . . .

The cop shrugged again, turned away and returned to his intersection. That would have been the end of it if the preacher hadn't followed him back to his post.

Disorderly conduct, like beauty, is in the eye of the beholder. Praying in front of a restaurant isn't against the law, but praying into a cop's ear while he's trying to direct traffic is. When your brain is saturated with the chemicals of schizophrenia, that's the kind of fine distinction you fail to make.

While remaining outwardly friendly, Richard nonetheless tried not to sit too close to the man. As a schizophrenic relapses, another sensitivity that vanishes is squeamishness about smells. Like most of Richard's new patients, the preacher desperately needed a bath.

But the best thing now was to get the man into isolation, so the chemical tides could ebb. Richard rose from the chair and beckoned for the patient to follow. The door with only one knob clicked softly behind them.

Richard led the man down the hallway to a door with a small, wire-reinforced glass window in it. He opened the door with his key and ushered the patient inside. There was a single bed, with a bare mattress. You can't hang yourself with a mattress.

It would help the preacher to have some time with himself. Psychiatrists saw the value of unstructured time long before the scientists began to theorize about how the brain revs up and dies down.

In that context, one of Richard's favorite brain scientists was an elder scientific statesman by the name of Dr. Paul McLean, who had a large laboratory complex up north of Washington, D.C. The laboratory was full of monkeys and lizards.

McLean said evolution had given man not one brain, but three. There was a lizard brain at the bottom, and on top of that there grew a mammal brain. Finally, superimposed on top of that, sat the cortex. Schizophrenia was a disease of the primitive brain, the lizard one.

Aeons ago the lizard brain evolved to handle life's more simple and brutal problems. It provided the dinosaur's ancestors with a sense of time, and a dislike for being eaten. It governed sex and territoriality. It told the creature when to go to sleep and when to wake up, when to get excited and when to bask in the sun.

Now, beneath the two more sophisticated brains, the lizard brain sits at the crossroads of the personality, directing and filtering information. The lizard brain is compelling, and it can make you hear voices and see things.

But the lizard is a dull creature, and can't maintain its interest without outside stimulation. Left alone, in an unmoving environment, the lizard's internal fires bank down and he ceases to move. A lizard, so deprived of stimulation, can sit without moving for hours.

The preacher will benefit from his stay in the seclusion room. In a few hours the lizard will calm down, the voices will cease and his real personality will begin to emerge.

Richard left the man sitting on the side of the bed, staring at the wall. He locked the door from the outside, and returned to his desk.

Now. Let's see.

He opened the preacher's file and searched through the report for a next of kin. The preacher had given the cops a woman's name.

Richard opened the telephone book and found a list of seven such names. He started calling at the top of the list. The last call connected him with the patient's mother.

As Richard had suspected, the patient had spent years in and out of mental institutions. Spring Grove State Hospital had given him a supply of Thorazine and released him three weeks ago. He probably quit taking the drug as soon as he hit the street.

Richard reassured the man's mother. Her son was okay, Richard said. He was personally seeing to it. After Richard hung up the telephone he reached into his desk drawer, removed the textbook he had been studying earlier and opened it to the marked page.

All this research about the brain and the mind bothered some of Richard's fellow counselors. Some of them seemed to resent the implication that they were chemical computers, for instance. And McLean's idea of the three-part brain, the "triune brain," he called it, often met resistance.

The lizard part of the triune brain theory bothered people. They could accept the mammalian brain, and recognize the emotions. Dogs feel love as well as people do, maybe better. But the lizard is a cold and amoral creature, a stimulus-response gizmo with all the love and compassion of a guided missile. The idea that a lizard was at the center of the psychological onion was simply unacceptable.

Richard was willing to concede that McLean's view of it was not particularly complimentary to the human species. Still, what new truth was ever pleasant? Evolution had been a comedown, too. But it led to modern biology and medicine.

Besides, Richard had been in the gutter, and it had made him wise. He looked carefully at the world around him, and he saw much in it to remind him of the lizard.

He remembered the dirty apartment. If he thought about it, which he did not like to do, he remembered it in stark detail. He could hear the flies buzzing. It was hot. He lay sprawled on the bed, staring at the ripped window screen.

He turned over. There was a woman beside him. She had a sore on her buttocks, and there were two flies feeding from it.

Richard never understood why, at that particular moment, he came to his senses. The flies had been there a long time, but only then did he connect them with filth.

He moved to wake the woman, then stopped. He sniffed the air. The odor was faint at first, until he realized it was there, and then it became overpowering. It came from the woman. He waved at the flies and they retreated from the sore—but not far. They weren't afraid of him.

The woman groaned in her sleep.

Richard sat up on the bed, wanting, wanting. He ached, he yearned, he craved. The heroin was on the dresser, but, for the moment, he didn't move toward it.

The smells grew stronger and stronger, enveloping him—the smell of the woman, of old shoes, of dirty socks, of the filthy diesel-tinged air that came in through the ripped screen.

The odor that was the worst of all was the one that he smelled last. It came from himself.

His mind spun. How many years had passed? The thought terrified him.

He sat on the bed for a long time, feeling the heroin craving pull against the terror. He knew the heroin would win this time, but he fought.

And that was something new.

It took a long time. Months. It was a daily fight, resisting the craving, fighting, failing, fighting, waiting as long as he could, stretching out the times between fixes, winning a little bit, capitulating, hating himself for his weakness, fighting again, winning, losing, winning, losing, winning, winning, winning . . .

His last fix was six years ago, and he had almost forgotten the warm pleasure of it. But he would never forget the smells of that apartment.

When it was all over he was broke, alone and hungry. He had stolen for heroin, but he would not steal for food. The car wash gave him a chamois and a plastic bottle of cleaner, and he spent each day caressing Cadillacs and Cordobas.

Later, the garbage-collecting job was better, and he got off early enough to go to night school.

The acute agony of breaking the addiction was over in a few weeks, but his mind did not clear so quickly. Before he started using drugs he had been a good student, but now the facts swam together, and he forgot things.

Doggedly, he studied harder, longer. He rose at three in the morning, walked to the corner, and when the garbage truck came, he swung himself up on its rear board. Time crawled. It seemed things would never get better.

But, slowly, they did.

Many of the memories of those old days, the addict days, were filed in dead storage. He didn't think of them much any more, except for the one thing that hung on, and on, and on.

The smell.

Sometimes it came to him, just a whiff, and he wanted to vomit.

It wasn't like the smell of the garbage truck, no, that was a garbage smell, an earthy smell of rotten fruit and moldy clothing. The smell that clung to Richard was another smell, a sick smell that seemed to waft out of his memory, a sharp smell of living death.

Soap and water would drive it away, temporarily.

While he was still fighting the craving, he learned the value of a shower. When he got his job with the Sanitation Department, he bought a kit to clean his fingernails and toenails, and a brush to scrub his back.

Each afternoon, as soon as he got home, he showered. An hour later, before leaving for school, he showered again.

He showered when he got home from school, before going to bed, and again when he got up. On Saturdays and Sundays he would sometimes stand in the shower for an hour, as the water turned from hot to tepid to cold. Still he stood there, shivering in the water, cleaning his fingernails and smelling the soap.

He made new acquaintances who didn't use heroin, and he kept his secret. He'd listen silently whenever his friends' conversation strayed to drugs, and their ignorance astonished him. They thought people who took drugs were evil and weak, no good, not like them.

They had no idea of the way drugs changed people, made them different, made the smells not matter, made them not care.

Sometimes, rarely now, he would get a yearning, an ache . . . and he pushed it down.

No. Never again.

No chemical would rule his life.

Slowly, as slowly as the returning self-respect, Richard realized that he could offer mental patients an understanding that others could achieve only at a distance, through the medium of books and training films.

Richard understood addiction and, by extrapolation, insanity. Therein lay a calling. As he helped himself, he could help others.

As his self-respect returned, a growing ambition to make something of himself led him to make inquiries, and his night classes took on a new direction. He would be a counselor.

First, he had to pass a state examination. He began to read everything he could find on the subject of addiction, mental illness and psychology.

He also needed a better job, one closer to his ambitions than dumping garbage cans.

One Sunday, after his second shower, he sliced a pear and an apple onto a plate and sat down to breakfast and the fat Sunday newspaper. He opened it to the want ads.

One of the job openings listed was for a counselor at a home for juvenile delinquents. The next day he applied. The supervisor was delighted to find a sober, intelligent, hardworking applicant.

That job lasted a year, while Richard studied and passed the state exam. Eventually he landed a job in the Mental Health Center as an intake counselor. Still, he continued to study. Eventually, he wanted to become a specialist, counseling victims of alcoholism, perhaps of drug addiction.

In the meantime, he had collected reasons to advance himself. He had found a woman, a marriage, and soon, very soon, a son or a daughter.

Tonight, even. Or tomorrow. From what the obstetrician said, it should have been four days ago. He tried not to think about it. The baby would come when it would.

In the meantime, he was ready. He had bought the cigars and opened a savings account for college. There was only ten dollars in it now, but there would be more. He had eighteen years.

His boy, by God, would go to college.

And that, to Richard, was one of the most wonderful feelings of all.

Richard forced his mind back to the textbook, and the baby vanished from his thoughts. He turned the page, then turned another. Occasionally, he underlined a passage.

It was three hours later, at almost 11 P.M., that his thoughts went back to the schizophrenic in isolation. He closed the book. Three hours should have been plenty of time.

The preacher must feel dirty, Richard thought. Hunger wouldn't come until later. The dirty feeling is first.

Richard put the envelope back in the book, closed it, and returned it to the top desk drawer. He collected the things he needed from the laundry room: one towel, one bar of soap, one toothbrush, a sample tube of toothpaste, a hand-me-down shirt and trousers from the prison system . . .

Richard wished he could give the man a fingernail brush, but the government didn't work that way. The government didn't understand the relationship between clean fingernails and healthy minds. Richard didn't really expect it to.

Richard peeked through the small window in the isolation room door. The man lay curled on the bed, his knees up, his eyes open. His mind, Richard knew, was adrift in the confusion that accompanies the waning of a chemical tide.

The patient sat up as the door opened.

Richard deposited the clean towel and clothing on the bed and hunkered down across from the schizophrenic. The man stared at him with a dull, burned-out look.

Feel better?

The eyes didn't waver. It was as though the man failed to hear.

Do you know where you are?

That got through.

Hospital. Hospital.

The man knew about hospitals. In response to Richard's gentle questions, he said he remembered not wanting to take his Thorazine. It was difficult for the patient to think. Richard saw the telltale signs of strain appearing around the man's eyes, and broke off the questioning.

Small things, at such a time, loom large. Shower?

The man comprehended the word "shower."

"Please," he said.

Richard walked slowly down the hallway, letting the man clutch his sleeve. It was important to do something positive, something for yourself. To deal with the chemicals in your head you had to know how to use the small things to your advantage.

It was something the Orientals talked about. Courage comes from within, but you can't search for it directly. You must look for it in the petals of a new rose, or in the rising steam of a hot shower.

"Thank you," the man said, clutching Richard's sleeve.

"Thank you, thank you, thank you, thank you sir."

As Richard learned about the human mind, he wasn't threatened by the idea that it was a chemical computer. That took nothing away from it. It was a computer, all right, but it was the most incredible computer imaginable.

No man-made computer would be stupid enough to addict itself. No man-made computer, having done so, would have had the inner resources to pull itself back up out of the stinking gutter.

If Richard could do it so could this man, and, with Richard's help, so could others.

CHAPTER
SEVEN

Dr. Salcman had been delighted to see the young girl with the pituitary tumor.

Well . . . delighted might be a poor word for it, since Cushing's syndrome was such a terrible thing. The mother and father brought the patient to his office, on the twelfth floor of University Hospital. They sat on the plastic chairs in front of Dr. Ducker's door, down the hallway, until Dr. Salcman got out of the operating room. They followed him into his office and sat stiffly on the state-issue chairs.

The poor girl sat hunched before him, sick and frightened. Her parents thrust a picture into his hand.

A petite teenager smiled back from the photograph. She had long black hair, clear skin and a fine mouth. Very pretty, definitely. Totally unlike the grotesque woman before him now.

They needn't have shown him the picture, really. The heavy breasts, the clumps of coarse black hair on her chest, the leathery skin, the acne, the beetle brow . . . they spoke eloquently. He knew as soon as he saw her.

Cushing's syndrome. Classic.

Wonderful. Wonderful because Dr. Salcman knew he could cure her. It was wonderful to cure someone.

Wonderful because the cure involved the elegant transphenoidal approach to the pituitary, at the bottom of the brain. Michael Salcman thought the transphenoidal approach, which went through the center of the face, was perhaps the most beautiful in modern neurosurgery. The operation left only a very tiny little hole in the skull, and no scar at all, but its effect was . . . magic.

The pituitary is a tiny thing no larger than a pea, but it's the master gland and it conducts the body's hormonal symphony. Acting on orders from the brain, for instance, the pituitary releases chemicals that are carried down in the bloodstream to regulate the orderly growth of cells.

Perhaps because the gland is so important, the forces of evolution have conspired to place it in one of the most protected parts of the body. It sits in a bony depression at the bottom of the cranial cavity, about three inches behind the bridge of the nose.

It was also nice, in an aesthetic sense, to treat a disease with such a rich and fascinating history. It had been Harvey Cushing, the first neurosurgeon, who had first understood the connection between the tiny, inaccessible pituitary and the gross facial features. And it had been Harvey Cushing himself who had designed the operation that Dr. Salcman would use.

It had all begun in 1896, when young Cushing arrived at Johns Hopkins, across town. Even as an apprentice surgeon he was audacious, the sort of young man who did things because, well . . . because others said they couldn't be done. One of the things that everybody believed couldn't be done was to operate on the brain. It had been tried, in desperate cases, but the patients always died.

Cushing read everything he could find on the brain. He concluded that the problem was the organ's delicacy—for one thing, when you touched it, tiny blood vessels ruptured. That caused swelling later, inside the confines of the skull. He also reasoned that if the tissue was that fragile, the plain water that surgeons used to keep their fields clear might also do harm. They should, he thought, use water with exactly the same salt content as human blood. It was little things, little things like that, that made all the difference.

Fellow surgeons warned him not to try it. His patients would die. For the most part they were right, but they weren't perfectly right, because an occasional patient recovered.

As time passed he thought of more and different ways to be careful. He reasoned that if he monitored pulse and breathing rate, he might get a warning when he got close to something . . . something deadly. The warning system worked so well that he started monitoring blood pressure too, and that worked even better. His successes launched a surgical specialty and set the stage for a second surgical giant, Walter Dandy, to earn Johns Hopkins Hospital a neurosurgical reputation that endures today.

That kind of reputation gave Hopkins an advantage that University of Maryland Hospital didn't have—that, and its protected status as a private, well-endowed institution. Cushing's modern heir, Dr. Donlin Long, didn't have to worry about the state legislature every year. Dr. Salcman's division head, Dr. Ducker, did.

The hospital in which Dr. Salcman operates is an example of a good state-run medical school. It trains most of the doctors who practice throughout Maryland, and its neurosurgical service has a growing reputation. At Maryland, the neurosurgeons like to point out that doctors from all over the country frequently bring their own wives and children to the University of Maryland Medical School when they need neurosurgery.

In fact, that was why the coarse-featured young woman with Cushing's syndrome had come all the way to Baltimore from her home in Central America. She had a relative who was a senior resident at the University of Maryland's Trauma Center.

Dr. Salcman examined the young woman carefully, and ordered a battery of tests that confirmed his diagnosis. He admitted the girl to the hospital and, allowing several days for the necessary tests, scheduled the transphenoidal for OR 11. He would talk to Dr. Ducker about getting Kay and Doris, and probably, yes, he would need OR 11 and the whole first team. It had to be a ballet. That was one of the things that was so beautiful about it.

Any day that began with a transphenoidal was a good day, and never mind the gusty Baltimore weather. He awoke with the upcoming operation on his mind, and it stayed there as he ran the razor over his stubbly face. It had to be in his mind, perfectly. He would be approaching the brain upside down, from underneath. He would have to think of the brain upside down today. Her right hemisphere would be on his left. Her left hemisphere would be on his right. In an emergency he wouldn't have time to stop and figure that out.

He came down the stairs, adjusting his tie, and his eyes found the bright red of a modern painting. He stared for a moment.

He had put the painting there, where it could cheer him in the mornings. On bad mornings, it helped. On a morning when he was going to do a transphenoidal, it was . . . wonderful.

An hour and a half later he stood in OR 11, in front of the X-ray board. One resident stood to his left and another to his right. A medical student stood on tiptoes behind.

Most of the films hanging on the X-ray board were standard CAT scans and skull X-rays, but one was different. It looked more like a black and white NASA photograph of some inhospitable, black-skied asteroid. The landscape was hilly and pitted with shallow holes.

It was, he told the younger men, a high-resolution X-ray taken across the bottom of the cranium, from ear to ear. The floor of the cranium is high, here, a shelf above the inner workings of the mouth and nose. The shelf supports the forebrain, then drops off in the rear to form a deep pit occupied by the lower brain.

Dr. Salcman touched the X-ray film with his finger, indicating a small, symmetrical crater in the bone. The residents leaned forward.

The difference between this depression and all the others is that this one, gentlemen, cradles the pituitary.

And notice—look closely—at the bottom of this depression, there's an even smaller depression. That is where the tumor has pressed against the bone and eroded it away. And that's where we're going to break through.

The residents peered at the tiny pit in the bottom of the somewhat larger tiny pit. The senior resident stepped back, momentarily, so the medical student could look.

Now, what that pit tells us is that the tumor's on the bottom of the pituitary. That's important, because if it's on the top then we can't go in from underneath. In that case, we'd have to go in through the temple, and push our way under the brain. The risk is higher that way.

In this case, we know it's on the bottom, so we can use the transphenoidal approach. An ear, nose and throat surgeon will do the first part, making the tunnel through the face. Then the neurosurgeons will take over.

A complicated operation. Complicated, but beautiful. A ballet. First team people working today, too. First team.

Dr. Salcman turned away from the X-ray board. Adroitly, the residents stepped aside. Fifteen feet away, across the operating room, the scrub nurse was readying her packages of sterile instruments and preparing to don her rubber gloves. The circulating nurse stood on her tiptoes to remove a package from the metal supply shelves that dominated one end of the room. The anesthesiologist sat by the patient, absorbed in filling out a form on his clipboard. Everyone knew exactly what to do. There was little talk.

The demands of brain surgery are not unlike those of war, insofar as they do not lend themselves to democracy. In Michael Salcman's operating room everything had to be perfect, absolutely perfect, and that meant somebody had to be in charge. That person, legally, morally and professionally, was Dr. Salcman.

He dominates his operating room the way a sea captain dominates his bridge, or a pilot his cockpit. Like the professors at Columbia who trained him, he is obeyed instantly, without hesitation.

Dr. Salcman likes his OR the way he likes it, perfect. He likes working with the first team, everyone thinking ahead, all precautions taken, each tool functioning, everything clean, silent, predictable, perfect.

Dr. Salcman likes it quiet, so it's quiet.

Somebody telling jokes might distract him, it might activate whatever part of his brain his mind uses to laugh, and for an instant he might forget that the brain was upside down today, and if he did that he might touch something that shouldn't be disturbed.

That doesn't apply to Dr. Salcman's jokes, of course. He knows when he can afford to laugh, and when he can't.

After turning away from the X-ray board, the neurosurgeon walked to the steel table where the patient lay, still conscious but very heavily sedated. Clasping his hand around hers, he bent over her.

"Everything is going to be all right," he said. "Everything is going to be all right, now."

Groggily, the girl nodded and raised her arm.

Dr. Salcman stood above her for a moment. She had been beautiful in the picture. She would be beautiful again.

Under Dr. Salcman's watchful eye, the team continued with its preparations. The anesthesiologist tended his beeping monitors, jumping dials and flashing lights. Everything synchronized. Perfect. Around the table, nurses and residents moved the surgical equipment into position.

When the ear, nose and throat surgeon arrived, Dr. Salcman took him to the X-ray board. For several minutes they talked in low tones. The ENT man traced a line across one of the X-ray films, from the girl's upper incisors to the middle of her head.

Then the two surgeons stood together, idly, watching the team work. The residents stood nearby, listening to the gossip.

Somewhere, a famous old surgeon had died and yeah, Michael had known him. Too bad. And did you read about the health care budget in last week's *Science*?

Did you hear that awful concert?

Dr. Salcman takes his music the same way he takes almost everything else, which is seriously.

By 7:30 A.M. the girl was unconscious and hidden by green drapes, the microscope was ready, the television monitor was working, and the ENT surgeon's specialized tools had been laid out.

The surgeon wore a headband, which held a lighted mirror with a hole drilled in it. Later he would pull it down and peer through the hole, but for now he simply stood above the girl. He looked down at her face, thoughtfully working the rubber surgical gloves around the base of his fingers.

Then he lifted her upper lip away from her teeth and held out his hand for the scalpel. The sharp steel cut upward, between lip and gum, from canine to canine. The surgeon stepped back, slightly, so that the resident could search for bleeders with the cauterizing tweezers.

The approach begun, the ENT surgeon pushed a long, sharp chisel up under the facial tissue, scraping the flesh away from the skull, forcing his way under the nose. He worked slowly and methodically. The chisel made an almost inaudible "snick, snick, snick" as it scraped against bone.

As the ENT surgeon worked his chisel between flesh and bone, the face began to change. It bulged upward, deforming. The girl's blood-flecked front teeth became visibly part of a skull.

As he pushed his way under the face, the surgeon paused to snip a small piece of cartilage from the gristly partition between the nostrils, called the septum. The scrub nurse took the little piece of rubbery tissue and carefully set it aside.

The cartilage shared a container with a small piece of fat. A neurosurgical resident had removed it from the girl's abdomen while the ENT man was scrubbing. Both bits of tissue would be needed later.

Finally the face was lifted clear and covered with a drape. Dr. Salcman looked over the ENT surgeon's shoulder as he shined his light through the nose hole in the skull, between the eye sockets, deep down into the center of the head. At the far end of the tunnel, the light fell on the ivory underside of the sphenoid sinus.

The scrub nurse handed the ENT surgeon a pair of long-handled nippers. Slowly, the surgeon lowered the nippers into the hole. The tiny jaws on the end maneuvered momentarily, then caught a protuberance of bone, tightened, and twisted.

There was an audible crunch as the fragile sinus floor yielded to titanium.

Dr. Salcman straightened and backed away. A resident waited a polite three seconds, then claimed the vacant vantage point.

The deepsink was in an open cul-de-sac off the main surgical hallway, between operating rooms eleven and twelve. Dr. Salcman mashed the foot pump and brown antiseptic soap squirted into his hands. Water roared from the faucet.

Upside down.

The brain would be upside down today.

Up is up and down is down but right is left and left is right.

The lather worked its way up his arm. Wash, rinse. Wash, rinse. Wash, rinse.

Think.

A neurosurgeon's brain must have the ability to conjure up a three-dimensional image of itself, to turn that image over and around and look at it from the bottom.

Dr. Salcman nodded absently to a passing heart surgeon. What could go wrong? A thousand things. Ten thousand. The one thing you didn't think of. And Big Red, of course.

In his head the model brain turned transparent, except for the network of arteries and veins. There were thousands of them, and they composed a fine net of interconnecting hoses, living hoses. The net was stiff, the hoses straining with the pressure. Dr. Salcman's brain thought about the vessels around the pituitary, reviewed them each, carefully, from underneath.

Satisfied, Dr. Salcman shifted his attention ever so slightly and the flesh of the brain appeared again, hiding the vessels. His mind moved on to other anatomy.

The changing mental map of the brain moved easily through Dr. Salcman's network of neurons. The electron paths were familiar. The landmarks all had familiar names, with histories and personal memories attached. With each year that passed, the mental map grew richer.

But the brain was also like Mark Twain's Mississippi. Maps were important, but the river changed every day. Dr. Salcman's image of the brain was as perfect as the ones in the anatomy books—but it wasn't exactly like the anesthetized brain awaiting him this morning. It wasn't exactly like any brain. Every brain was unique.

And each was, in its own unpredictable way, dangerous. If an approach like this was a ballet, it was also a balancing act, even a bullfight. Like a bullfight, there was danger. More people died in neurosurgical operating rooms than in bullrings, by far.

A ballet was more aesthetically pleasing to Michael Salcman. Or even baseball. Baseball, in fact, had a lot going for it. As a child in New York he had collected baseball cards, he had played . . .

Not very well, unfortunately. The tilted pelvis saw to that. The tilted pelvis pretty well ensured that he would never be a great baseball player. But on the other hand, out of adversity, polio had given him a commitment.

His foot found the pump, on the floor, and more brown soap squirted into his hands.

He had been only five, but even then he knew that polio was a paralyzing disease. He knew his parents were deathly afraid of it, because it was often fatal. They'd told him to stay out of the park, not to go running in the summer's heat, and he'd disobeyed.

The doctor had looked down at him, and told him the truth.

Even at five, and ill, Michael grasped that the doctor, in telling him the truth, had shown him respect.

After that, he lay in bed, paralyzed, and waited to die.

But he hadn't. The doctor had given him his life back. He didn't understand, then, that the doctor was unable to influence the course of the disease. All Michael knew was that the doctor cared for him, and he didn't die. He watched the man with awe.

Michael would be a doctor. The ambition imprinted itself onto the boy's mind and fueled his natural curiosity. With the help of tutors, the recovering boy studied to catch up with his classmates, and with great effort and encouragement from his mother, he succeeded.

As grade school ended, his brush with death receded into the past, leaving only a slight limp—and an unusually well-developed perception of his mission in life.

He would be a doctor.

It took many years before he knew exactly what kind of doctor he would be, but when the time came, the choice was natural and compelling. As a medical student he was drawn inexorably toward the brain, the fascinating brain, the target organ of polio. In the end, there would be no question. Michael Salcman would be a neurosurgeon.

As he grew, his curiosity was focused by his ambition. He was an excellent student. He finished high school at age sixteen, and immediately enrolled in Boston University's six-year medical school program. At age twenty-two, he would be a doctor and a scientist, entrusted to work at the National Institutes of Health laboratories near the nation's capital.

There, as part of the effort to attach artificial eyes and ears directly to the brain, Dr. Salcman concentrated on one of the most exacting techniques in neurosurgery—implanting electrodes into the living brains of laboratory animals.

Before his stay in Washington was finished, he had trained himself to use electrodes so tiny and delicate that he could place one in an individual brain cell. The technique required consummate skill, but when done properly it allowed him to listen in on the neuronal partyline conversations of a single cell.

The experience reinforced everything he already knew about brain surgery. He had to be perfect, or the cell he stuck the sensor into would die. He had to be perfectly clean or the animal would become infected, the neuron would die, and the party line would shut down.

It was wonderful training for a neurosurgeon-to-be. Now, many years later, Dr. Salcman washed his forearms and reviewed the decisions he would need to make if anything went wrong.

Something could always go wrong, but if you were good enough, and careful enough, and had prepared your fallback positions well enough, there were ways to deal with the something, the whatever, and win.

Not always, of course. Nobody wins always. And when you lose, patients die—a day later, perhaps, or two.

At least Dr. Salcman had never lost a patient on the table, never had one die beneath his hands. Sometimes he would brag a little about that, but cautiously, because, God help him, he tempted fate every time he said it . . . but he was proud of the fact.

And if the day ever came, and he lost a patient on the table, well, that day was part of the unthinkable future. Today was today, a magic day, a great day for a transphenoidal. There would be no death in OR 11 today.

His scrub ritual complete, Dr. Salcman held his hands over the sink, to drip. A minute later, in the OR, the scrub nurse tied the straps on his sterile gown.

Gowned and gloved, the neurosurgeon returned one more time to the X-ray board. His eyes searched for the tiny crater in the bone, and the tinier crater inside it.

It was 9:35 by the time Dr. Salcman and the senior resident swung the microscope into place, and the most dangerous phase of the operation began. Dr. Salcman looked through the eyepieces, touching the electrical control buttons through sterile plastic. The hum of the focusing motor was barely audible.

The microscope was a very good one. Michael Salcman wouldn't have it any other way.

But at the moment . . . it wasn't right. Something wasn't right. The neurosurgeon frowned.

"This thing's not aimed correctly," he finally said to the resident. Methodically, he explained to the resident that if the microscope wasn't adjusted perfectly, the surgeon would have to compensate, and compensating would make him more awkward.

That meant less perfect, which meant something was more likely to happen.

The resident listened in silence as he helped adjust the microscope. He'd heard the lecture before, and he would hear it again. Before he becomes certified by the American College of Neurosurgeons, such truths will visit him in his sleep.

Now. Let's try again.

Dr. Salcman peered into the eyepieces again and touched the power-focus button. A crystal-clear image of bone appeared on the monitor. It was crisscrossed with tiny vessels.

Perfect. See? Just like that.

You have to remember, every minute, that you're beneath the brain and looking up. Up is forward, down is back, right is left and left is right.

The circulating nurse touched a wall switch and the operating room lights died, their filaments glowing briefly in the dark. The anesthesiologist's dials and lights glowed softly. The miscroscope had its own headlights that shined down under the girl's face and illuminated the floor of the cranium.

Dr. Salcman lectured as he worked.

You need the microscope adjusted perfectly. Remember, errors compound. Something small goes wrong and then what you do to correct it doesn't work perfectly, and things get worse, and if you're not very calm, that's when you touch something that should not be disturbed.

Teaching is important to Dr. Salcman. All the great neurosurgeons taught. It helped keep them on their toes, and it extended their influence down through the generations. The resident might look tired, and he might indeed have heard the lecture before, but it is a hard world and the resident is grateful for each of his teacher's words. At least, that's the way it had been for Dr. Salcman.

When he finished his work at NIH and asked for a neurosurgical residency at Columbia University, there were more than one hundred and fifty other applicants. He was thankful to be one of the three accepted, and he kept his mouth shut, and his eyes open.

He might not have appeared grateful at the time, but deep down beneath the bruised ego and the overwork, he knew that there were truths that must be engraved into a neurosurgeon's brain.

He listened and he watched. As he progressed, he took the best that each professor had to offer, and now his own approach was an amalgam of them all. The job of passing it on was one he took seriously.

Dr. Salcman's voice rose slightly as he changed the subject and addressed the entire operating room team.

"You know what diplomacy is?" he asked.

He waited for answers, but since he had addressed no one in particular, he didn't get any.

Beep, beep, beep, beep, went the heart monitor. The girl's heart rate was steady, seventy beats a minute.

"It's the ability to juggle four balls in the air while keeping your own intact," he finally said, answering himself.

The resident groaned.

The second hand on the clock swung around, and around again.

Dr. Salcman looked down the main barrels of the microscope while the resident used the side eyepieces. The tiny circle of light from the instrument's headlight was the brightest illumination in the room. The television monitor duplicated the surgeon's view down the long tunnel behind the girl's face.

The senior neurosurgeon called the resident's attention to a tiny ridge of bone in the center of the microscope's field.

Right there.

That ridge marks the spot.

If you make the hole right there, exactly there, you will come up through the floor of the cranium, right under the pituitary, right where the tumor is, exactly.

Now. You do it.

The resident took a deep breath and moved over to the main barrels of the microscope. Dr. Salcman moved to the side 'scope, to watch, instruct, coach and assist. The resident will get the practice, but Michael Salcman will make the decisions.

After adjusting the main 'scope to suit his eyes and his height, the resident scanned the wall of bone at the end of the microscope.

Right there.

Exactly. Right there.

The resident held out his right hand and the scrub nurse handed him a long instrument with a chisel point. Without moving his eyes away from the microscope, he moved the instrument toward the incision.

Dr. Salcman guided the resident's hand until the end of the chisel swam into view.

The resident lowered it to the bone, and put his hand out for the mallet.

He moved the mallet softly.

Tap.

He pulled the chisel back and examined the tiny chip he had made. Then he placed the chisel against the bone again.

The microscope amplified every motion. Each time he changed the chisel's position, it seemed to swim ponderously across the microscopic field of view. It shuddered with the slightest motion of the resident's hand.

Tap.

Tap.

Each tap knocked away a tiny piece of bone, a microscopic piece of bone. The object was to chip around the edges of a square until, finally, that square fell free.

The skull was very thin there, almost like an eggshell, Dr. Salcman lectured.

Don't shatter it, don't break through accidentally.

Tap. Tap. Tap-tap.

Easy.

Tap.

Careful. Careful, careful.

You can't push on the brain.

The resident's movements were slow and deliberate. The tension was thick. The chisel moved aside, allowing the surgeons to inspect the damage. Then the instrument moved back again, found its spot.

Tap. Tap-tap.

Careful, careful.

The chisel was huge.

Tap, pause, tap, pause, tap, pause.

Too much pressure and the skull might cave inward, pressing on the tumor, and the tumor would press on the pituitary, and the patient would . . . do poorly, very poorly indeed.

The resident's face was a study in concentration.

Tap.

Tap-tap.

Tap.

The clock hands moved slowly. Dr. Salcman was silent.

Finally, a tiny square of bone came free—or seemed to. But when the resident attempted to gently tease it away from the brain with a tiny hook, something . . . caught.

Disengage!

There was a sharp bite to Dr. Salcman's voice. The resident obeyed, instantly.

You've got to be gentle, see?

"It *wants* to come out. You tease it and it comes to you. If it doesn't come and you have hold of it, then let go. Don't pull, because it might be attached to something that shouldn't be moved."

The resident tried again.

"Yes," Dr. Salcman said. "That way."

Gently. Carefully. You have to plan every action, never move an instrument unless you've thought it through first. If you made a mistake down this tube, you'd never recover the situation.

The resident worked with the hook, gently prying at the square trapdoor of bone between him and the brain. Not really prying, of course, because that was like pulling, more teasing at the bone, cajoling, beckoning.

Finally, with tortuous slowness, the bone flap came free. The resident fished it out of the hole and handed it to the nurse on the tip of one gloved finger. She grasped it with forceps, and discarded it.

The resident stared down the microscope. Through the tiny square hole in the underside of the skull, he could see the leathery dura mater, the mother membrane, the outer level of the meninges.

Both surgeons peered down the microscope, examining.

The nurse put a long, thin instrument in the resident's hand, and Dr. Salcman took his eyes away from the eyepieces long enough to guide the resident's hand down the tunnel. That's one of the things he tried to teach the residents. How to assist. Guide the surgeon's hand into the hole. Help him until he can see the instrument through the microscope.

To the naked eye, the instrument looked sharp. Under the microscope its tip was smooth and rounded. It touched the dura and pushed, no, not pushed, gently touched, caressed, tested. Under the microscope, the dura seemed the consistency of thick white leather. It resisted the instrument, giving way slowly.

Careful.

Dr. Salcman guided the resident's hand as it lifted the probe from the tunnel, then guided it back in with a new instrument.

A knife swam into view on the monitor. Strain showed around the resident's eyes as he struggled to hold it steady, perfectly steady.

The knife touched the dura, and carefully, carefully, began to move.

No.

Dr. Salcman's voice changed pitch.

No, no, no, not that way, not that way, *not that way!*

Under the microscope, blood flowed slowly, leisurely, onto the field.

No. You cut it the wrong way. You've got to know that the dura contains wide channels for blood drainage. They aren't even veins, really, just wide, collapsed pouches. You have to remember that the pouches all run in one direction. If you cut across one, you can burn it closed with the electric tweezers and that's that. No problem. But if you split one lengthwise, the bleeding mouth of the wound will be too big to seal.

And now look what you've got!

And the hole you're working in is so small, and so confining. If you can't get the bleeding stopped you have to retreat. You can't continue.

And if you can't continue, you've lost. And you've failed the patient. And you've ruined . . . and you've absolutely ruined a beautiful operation.

Both surgeons looked with dismay at the dark blood oozing from the dura.

As Dr. Salcman's part of the operation had gotten under way, the scrub nurse had spent several minutes arranging the wires and tubes that led to the micro-bipolars, one of neurosurgery's most versatile instruments. The bipolars consisted of a pair of electric cauterizing tweezers. Dr. Salcman's bipolar tweezers were an even fancier model, with a suction device built into one tong. Now, when the resident called for the bipolars, she was ready.

As the resident lowered the bipolars into the tunnel, Dr. Salcman guided his hand.

In the microscopic field the bipolars moved toward one of the bleeding edges of the meninges. The instrument caught the oozing edge, but then it slipped free. The resident concentrated, and tried again. This time he caught it more firmly and the electricity sizzled through the tissue, forming a little rivet of burned flesh. Briefly, blood oozed back over the field, and then the suction cleared it.

For a while, as the resident worked to seal the edges of the hole, Dr. Salcman gave advice from the side microscope. Then they were orders. In a few minutes he stepped back.

Change places.

The resident seemed relieved.

Dr. Salcman took his place, touched the adjusting buttons, then stared thoughtfully down the barrels of the microscope. His hand reached, almost absently, for the bipolars. The resident, now at the side 'scope, touched Dr. Salcman's hand to help him guide the instrument down the tunnel.

Now there were no jokes.

In the microscopic field, they fought the battle to stop the bleeding.

Irrigation.

The water swirled like a tidal wave through the microscopic topography, turning to red as it mixed with blood.

Suction, please.

The ocean moved, whirlpooling, toward the suction tip of the bipolars. For a moment, the view was clear. The eye could see the bleeding wound.

Seizing that moment, Dr. Salcman's hand moved, quickly but not too quickly, gently . . .

On the monitor screen, the bipolar tweezers darted toward the bleeder and expertly clamped the central section shut. Cauterizing electricity sizzled through the dura mater.

Irrigation. Suction. More irrigation, please.

Zzzzzzzt, went the bipolars.

The surgeon worked quickly, his eyes pressed to the microscope. His hands barely moved, but each movement was greatly magnified. The bleeding was slow, but constant. There was sweat on the resident's neck.

Suction.

Irrigation.

Zzzzzzt.

The minutes passed, and the heart monitor beeped rhythmically in the background. Suction, irrigation, grab the bleeder, push the switch. Suction, irrigation, grab the bleeder, push the switch. Finally, the crevice was welded shut and the resident took a deep breath.

Dr. Salcman stepped back and flexed his shoulders. The day was saved, but his buoyant mood did not return immediately. The incident had marred what was supposed to be a perfect operation.

Now he would have to keep one part of his mind on the bleeder during the rest of the operation. He wouldn't dare disturb it. He would always have to know exactly where it was and exactly what to do if it broke open again.

He stepped back to the microscope and, taking the knife, proceeded to finish opening the dura. As the flap came away, the tissue behind it glistened in the headlights. The scrub nurse stared at the monitor, her hands hovering above the instruments that she thought the surgeon would ask for next.

Dr. Salcman stared at the little square of exposed pituitary tissue. Right in the middle, dead in the middle, was a tiny, slightly discolored speck. The tumor.

Instantly, his good humor returned.

He had planned the operation perfectly, absolutely perfectly.

The tumor was exactly where he had predicted it would be. He had come up right under it.

Despite the bleeder, then, it was going to be a beautiful operation.

The surgeon called for the microsuction device, a thin metal tube attached to a suction hose. The nurse had anticipated correctly, and it was quickly in his hand.

With the sucker, he could tease those discolored cells away.

The nurse watched the television monitor. The sucker, large under the strong magnification, moved briefly, hesitantly, above the tumor. Slowly, reconnoitering almost, carefully, it settled, touched . . . and backed away.

Never pull.

Plead. Cajole. Touch and jump away. Never mind the minutes. Each touch disturbs thousands of cells, sets up shock waves that move through the tissue, that might tear a neuron and disconnect something.

The sucker nudged at the tumor. It was right next to the little speck of cells that control water metabolism. The heart monitor beeped steadily.

Careful.

Dr. Salcman teased at the tumor, brushed at it, beckoned at it, and a few cells drifted off its surface and came to him, jamming the orifice of the sucker. He brought the instrument out, transferred the dot of tissue to the taut rubber surface of his index finger, and passed it to the scrub nurse. The scrub nurse put it in a container and gave it to the circulating nurse. The circulating nurse took it and walked quickly, almost ran, out of the operating room and toward the surgical pathology laboratory.

Dr. Salcman stood with his sterile hands extended in front of him, waiting. For a moment, no one spoke. Then Dr. Salcman broke the silence.

"The trouble with the operating room," he said, "is that there isn't any wood to knock on."

Dr. Salcman had told the girl and her parents that the tumor probably wasn't cancerous, and he would be very surprised if it was. Surprised, but not exactly astounded. Now, before proceeding, he had to know.

In fact, all tumor operations had this built-in pause, waiting for the moment of truth. Was it a primary malignant tumor, and had it grown to the stage where it had probably seeded itself throughout the body? Or was it a secondary cancer, a seedling from something growing malevolently in the lungs or gut?

In this case, Dr. Salcman didn't expect either answer. This kind of tumor was more like a wart, and it did its damage not by consuming the tissue around it, but by exerting a gentle pressure. Tumors of the pituitary were almost never cancerous.

Usually, waiting for the pathology report was a grim business for Dr. Salcman, a depressing business. Most of his patients had glioblastoma multiforme, the most malignant brain tumor of all.

And it was depressing. Dr. Salcman didn't kid himself about that, didn't try to sublimate it. It was damned depressing, when so many of your patients died. That had been one of the first things he'd told Dr. Ducker, the day Dr. Ducker revealed what was in store for him.

Glioblastoma multiforme.

Messy. A killer. An inexorable killer. Six months from diagnosis, usually.

Depressing.

But, as Dr. Ducker pointed out, somebody had to do it. And nobody was doing anything much for glioblastoma multiforme victims, after all. Nobody wanted to get involved. It was too damned depressing.

But . . . it's also depressing to have all your patients die.

Tom Ducker had commiserated with him, all right, but he hadn't withdrawn the . . . what? They weren't exactly orders, or precisely a request . . .

Dr. Salcman fought, briefly, with himself.

What Dr. Ducker had said about how somebody had to help those people, that much was accurate. Rather horribly so. Horribly for the patients, and horribly for Dr. Salcman, who, unfortunately, perhaps, knew his duty.

It wasn't an order, really. It was a . . . charge.

Desperately, Dr. Salcman negotiated. If he agreed to do glioblastoma multiforme, could he have his pick of the other tumors? The more interesting ones?

The curable ones?

If he had to take the glioblastoma multiformes, could he have the acoustics, too, the hearing-nerve tumors? And the pineals? And, of course, the pituitary tumors?

If he could do a few transsphenoidals, it would help.

Dr. Ducker considered the proposal, and judged it fair.

Now Dr. Salcman stood in OR 11, surrounded by the first team, exchanging greetings with the pathologist who stood in the doorway, a mask held over his face with one hand.

"Basophil microadenoma," the pathologist intoned. Dr. Salcman smiled beneath his mask. Noncancerous. As predicted. Beautiful.

Dr. Salcman moved back to the microscope. His hand went out for the sucker.

The tumor was only a tiny thing, much smaller than the tip of his little finger. The sucker moved across it, time and time again, and the tumor slowly abraded. Soon, the abnormal tissue was gone. After washing the field with water and examining the tissue carefully, Dr. Salcman stood and switched places with the resident.

At the neurosurgeon's request, the scrub nurse produced the pieces of tissue saved from earlier, the tiny bit of cartilage from the nose and the chunk of fat from the abdomen.

The resident cut off a small piece of the fat and grasped it firmly between the jaws of a long-handled instrument. Under Dr. Salcman's critical eye he moved the fat into the microscopic field and approached the square hole in the bone.

Careful, careful, Dr. Salcman instructed the resident. Not that way, not that way, yes, that way, steady.

Steady.

Gently, the resident tucked the fat through the rectangular hole in the bottom of the skull. It would cushion the brain tissue and help seal the hole.

Next, Dr. Salcman told the operating team, they would cut a square of cartilage just a little bit bigger than the hole and, bending it just so, would work it through the opening. It would lie there, on the floor of the cranium, like a piece of plywood over a construction pit. Eventually, the bone would heal.

It took several minutes to trim the cartilage to the exact size and shape. The process involved several trips down into the tunnel, to hold the cartilage beside the hole for comparison.

After several fittings and trimmings, the square of cartilage met the resident's approval. After a few more, it met Dr. Salcman's.

Now, bending it just so . . .

Dr. Salcman coached from the side 'scope.

If you bend it just right, no, no, not that way. This way. Over there.

Try it the other way . . . try it again . . . careful. Easy, now. The best way to operate on the pituitary gland, as on the brain, is not to touch it. Don't ever pull on anything. If you don't know where you are, stop.

The cartilage hesitated, and slipped in.

"Beautiful," said Dr. Salcman.

The resident sighed deeply. It would be over quickly, now.

The rest of the fat was used to pack the sphenoid sinus and then get out, retreat, let sleeping dogs lie, don't touch the bleeder, get out, flee with your victory, and let the ENT man stitch the front of her face back on.

When it was over, the ENT surgeon left. Dr. Salcman stood back, stripped off his gloves and watched as the anesthesiologist administered an antidote for the anesthetic.

The patient moved, groggily, painfully. Already her face was turning blue with bruises.

But they would heal.

Dr. Salcman bent over the bed. "It's all over now," he said. "Everything went perfectly. You're going to be just fine."

Dr. Salcman was ebullient, making jokes for the benefit of the resident as they followed the patient's bed out into the hallway.

And it was a good day.

A great day, already, and it wasn't even noon.

God, it was wonderful to cure someone!

CHAPTER
EIGHT

TONY MASTROSTEPHANO'S COMPUTER WAS A REMARKABLE THING. ITS component parts occupied row upon row of metal cabinets, all linked together by a complex network of cables beneath the floor. The air was carefully filtered, and since the computer had a tendency to overheat, the temperature was kept just slightly below the human comfort level. The humans who tended the computer kept sweaters in their desks.

On occasion, Tony's duties required him to guide visitors through the computer room. He usually enjoyed it, and the people were usually impressed. He always let them stand a few minutes, uninterrupted, to soak up the atmosphere. Magnetic disks turned, tapes advanced, printers chattered, technicians moved purposefully about, the false floor bouncing a little with each footstep.

Later he might explain that they didn't actually see the computer. The computer itself was almost an abstract thing, something you had to imagine, like you had to imagine a soul, or an atom. The thing was no more tangible than a set of changing circuits and flowing electrons. What the visitors saw was the peripheral stuff, the equipment that fed information to the computer and then extracted it.

The computer worked all the time, of course, and three shifts of servants tended it. During the day it fed on information sent in by satellite computers in the company's branch offices. It stored the input in bursts of electricity, to mull over while the salesmen and actuaries slept. In the morning it told its master, an insurance firm, exactly how much had to be paid to the woman in Tampa who became a widow yesterday.

It was the kind of huge, number-crunching computer that could be made, with a little hyperbole, to seem downright spooky. Tony could make it seem so, if he sensed that was what the visitor wanted to hear.

But he himself, as master technician, was privately unimpressed. It was very big, but also very dumb.

It couldn't tell you when to bluff in a poker game, it couldn't tell "Rock Lobster" from Beethoven, and it didn't even know enough to look forward to payday. It couldn't do anything you didn't program into it, and programming was no Einsteinian feat—Tony hired and fired programmers.

In Tony's view, the most wondrous thing about the computer was that it kept him and his technicians in potatoes and, occasionally, lobster.

To Tony, the visitors were far more interesting than what they were ogling. People were interesting.

Tony loved his job, which was managing people who tended computers, and he was very good at it. He motivated them when they were lazy, counseled them when they had marital problems, traded stories with them at lunch.

Some said there weren't any basic differences between a brain and a computer, and in a sense that was true. But while the machine could be cursed at, it couldn't curse back and didn't care, either way. Tony's people had personalities, and the dullest of them was far more interesting than the smartest and fastest computer.

It wasn't the sort of thing that Tony thought about very much, but he acted on it every day. He ignored the computer, for the most part, leaving his technicians to worry about its care. His wife called him a workaholic, and he confessed he was, but it wasn't the computer that brought him to work so enthusiastically. It was the people.

Of course, he'd had cause to observe recently, the computer did have one distinct advantage over man. It didn't have headaches.

The headaches had come on very slowly, and for a while he hadn't even noticed. When he did notice, he managed to ignore it. Later, when it wouldn't be ignored, he learned to smother it in aspirin. He didn't even think about staying home, and he didn't believe in complaining. Complaining never helped anything. Besides, he had work to do.

But he'd been slowing down lately. It helped to find a quiet corner, sit down, close his eyes and massage his temples.

Then one day even that didn't help. The pain came out and enveloped him, crushed him, and he couldn't think about the computers, or the tapes, or the programmers. He couldn't think about anything but the pain.

Later he remembered that someone took him to his car, and he remembered every agonizing bump in the road between Valley Forge and Audubon, where he lived. Then there were his wife's gentle hands, placing cold towels on his forehead. There were clean sheets and a dark bedroom.

Jean left him alone in the dark and went to the kitchen, although there was nothing to do. She leaned against the countertop.

She was shaken. If Tony had actually allowed himself to be brought home, it was serious. She resolved that her husband would go to a doctor. Not next week. Tomorrow.

He didn't even put up a fuss, which was unlike him.

The physician examined Tony very thoroughly and found nothing wrong. He didn't appear surprised. As a rule, he said, patients who complain of headaches have no identifiable physical problems.

Headaches were usually caused by tension in the scalp, squeezing the nerves there. Stress, perhaps. Or fatigue. God knows what, but nothing the doctor could fix.

Given time, it'd probably fix itself.

The doctor wrote a prescription for a painkiller and slid it across the desk. Tony folded it, put it in his shirt pocket, and dropped it off at the drugstore on his way to work.

Jean was not satisfied. The doctor hadn't called Tony a malingerer, but Jean had understood by his manner that he thought he might be.

In this case he was wrong, she was sure of it. Her husband was not a malingerer. She wished he was.

A sense of foreboding settled over her.

The painkillers worked for a few days, but then there was a knock on the door. When Jean opened it, there was Tony again, in the middle of the day. Again, one his employees was with him.

They went back to the doctor.

This time the physician was frankly puzzled. He looked at the chart. Tony Mastrostephano's record didn't reflect a tendency to make things up, and his wife was being, well, insistent.

Maybe it was a sinus condition.

Maybe his membranes were swelling and blocking the sinuses, which can cause pressure to build. That can result in absolutely incredible headaches.

The doctor gave Tony and his wife the name of a good ear, nose and throat specialist.

But in a few days they were back, both of them. The report said the specialist had checked out everything in the ear, nose and throat bailiwick, and found nothing remarkable. No sinus condition.

The doctor was at a loss, but experience had taught him that Nature was wonderful. Given time, most things cured themselves. Otherwise, doctoring would be a very depressing profession.

The doctor wrote a prescription for a stronger painkiller. Tony dropped it off on his way to work.

He had the headaches all the time now, but he learned that he could work around them. He could think of the computer, and the air-filtration system for the computer room, and the programmer's new baby. Only occasionally would he give up, go home, and lie perfectly still in the darkened bedroom.

Tony, perhaps, could have survived that way for a long while, but Jean couldn't. Each time Tony came home early, her certainty increased. Something was wrong.

Again, she took her husband to the doctor.

Okay, the doctor said. There is one more option.

He gave them the name of a neurologist at Bryn Mawr Hospital, just outside Philadelphia. Jean drove, trying to avoid bumps.

Jean recited her story to the neurologist. When she was done, he removed a large safety pin from his lapel, opened it, and used it to prick the skin on Tony's forearm.

Do you feel that?

Yes.

How about that?

Yes.

The specialist tested the skin on various parts of Tony's body. He moved a finger in front of Tony's eyes, and Tony followed it. Tony stood up, bent his knees, and stood on one foot.

Then he led Tony to a straight chair, sat him down and instructed him to stare straight ahead. The doctor bent over him, peering into his eyes with a lighted instrument.

The light swept over his retinas while the doctor, looking through the ophthalmoscope's lenses, searched this visible extension of the brain for signs of swelling.

The neurologist's trained eye focused immediately on the swollen optic disk, and he made a noncommittal noise.

Then he stood up, walked to his desk and picked up the telephone. Tony and Jean waited while he arranged for a test of some sort at Bryn Mawr. After he hung up, the neurologist leaned on his desk and asked Tony if he'd ever heard of a CAT-scanner.

Vaguely.

A CAT-scanner was a sophisticated kind of X-ray machine that takes pictures of the inside of the head. And it doesn't hurt, not at all.

You lie on a table, and it takes your picture. They'll be ready for you as soon as you arrive, and when you're finished, come back here.

At the hospital, the CAT-scan attendants took Tony's clothes and gave him a gown. Then they helped him up onto a table, with his head at the mouth of a big metal doughnut. As he had been instructed, Tony lay perfectly still. The table moved forward, centimeter by centimeter. After each movement, something in the doughnut clicked.

Then Tony put on his clothes, met Jean in the waiting room, and went with her back to the neurologist's office. Almost immediately the neurologist ushered them into his office.

Images of Tony's brain were already hanging on the glowing X-ray board. Each sheet of film was about the size of a large manila envelope, and was subdivided into four images. Jean could see that each image was a "slice" through a human brain. Tony's brain.

The tumor was the big white fuzzy spot in the left temporal lobe, over the left ear. Once it was pointed out, Jean could see it clearly. It wasn't subtle.

The doctor explained carefully, directing his voice at Tony. Jean listened, numb.

There are only two kinds of cells in the brain, the gray ones that process information and the white ones that take care of the gray ones. The gray ones never grow into tumors because they can't reproduce. But the white ones can. Once in a while, in a rare while, they turn malignant.

Jean's mind refused to process the word "malignant," but she stored it for contemplation later. The phrase "less than a year" made no sense either, and was cataloged as well.

The shadow on the CAT scan was very characteristic, the doctor was saying. An operation could extend life, but the tumor always came back. The doctor said he had already made arrangements for Tony to check into the hospital.

Immediately, he said. Today. Right now.

Tony stood slowly, fiddling with the zipper on his coat. Jean took his arm and led him out. Later, she would not remember the short walk to the hospital.

"Mastrostephano," she told the admitting clerk. "M-a-s-t-r-o-s-t-e-p-h-a-n-o."

Jean dug through her purse for the insurance card. There were blanks to fill out and questions to answer.

Tony was polite, quiet, distant. He let Jean handle it.

When the paperwork was finished she went upstairs with him and fussed while he put on the hospital-issue nightshirt.

The next thing to do, she decided methodically, was to go home, tell their eighteen-year-old son, get Tony's pajamas and pack some toilet articles.

She'd be back soon, she promised.

It was dark outside, drizzly. The wipers skipped across the window, streaking.

Jean knew the neighborhood well and, as she drove, her mind went back to the neurologist's office.

A tumor.

Malignant.

A year.

Tony's face hadn't changed expression. It was as though nothing had been said.

Jean knew how his mind worked. She knew with the experience of twenty-five years of marriage, knew from the insights of mature love, knew, without a doubt, that Tony hadn't comprehended a thing.

A year.

If Tony didn't want to understand, then she wouldn't try to make him. It would be her responsibility.

A year. A year is a long time, if it's a happy year. Could it be more than a year? Might a cure be found in that year? She drove automatically, her mind awash with conflicting hopes and dreads. Suddenly her attention snapped back to the glistening road.

Where was she?

The car slowed, drifted through an intersection, and stopped. The wipers slapped rhythmically from side to side.

Paul McLean says men and women have lizard brains, and in that, they are no different from reptiles. They have emotional, mammalian brains as well, as do opossums and cows.

But superimposed on those, primates have yet another brain, the cerebral cortex. The cortex is most dramatically developed in the human species, where it reaches the size of half a cantaloupe.

The cortex blesses man with the ability to think ahead, to scheme, to plan, to build. But it is also a curse. With his cortex, man, and man alone, can foresee death.

And man is the only creature that cries.

Lost and alone, Jean slumped over the steering wheel, sobbing.

CHAPTER
NINE

DR. LONG'S CALENDAR AT JOHNS HOPKINS WAS, IN SOME RESPECTS, THE most important document in his neurosurgical kingdom. The calendar was kept by Fran Crow, who sat at a desk immediately beside the door to the chairman's inner office. Technically Fran was a secretary, but the responsibility for the calendar elevated her to a higher role as judge and arbiter.

The calendar was a large, softbound book that opened out to display the entire month. For months ahead, its pages were packed with Fran's neat handwriting.

Each entry represented a hard-won compromise between the conflicting demands of rounds, surgery, salesmen, scientists, conference chairmen, visiting firemen, reporters, residents, public officials, attorneys and pain patients. Dr. Long was very well-known in pain.

Visitors came at precise times. Sometimes they had to wait briefly beside Fran's desk, where they could, if they liked, examine Dr. Long's collection of exotic plants on the window ledge. Fran couldn't offer them a chair, because there was none to offer.

When Dr. Long was free, Fran escorted the visitors through his door, and when their time was up, she escorted them out again. Dr. Long's life was very precisely choreographed, and last-minute changes could blow down the whole house of cards.

So when Fran looked up from her typewriter and saw Dr. Murray standing politely beside her desk, she felt a vague apprehension. When it came to the calendar, Dr. Murray had Top Priority.

Yes sir, she said, reaching for the book.

The twelfth?

She looked with dismay at the full calendar.

The twelfth. Yes sir. She made a notation, then underlined it.

Yes sir. She would put Dr. Long on alert that day.

After Dr. Murray left, Fran stared for a moment at the book, ar-

ranging her options. Of course, an alert didn't mean he would actually
be called. Whatever was going on in the OR might turn out to be
simpler than expected, and there would be no call.

She would have to play it by ear.

Across the office, Dr. Long's other secretary, Pat Diniar, was on the
telephone. She was being very firm with a pain patient. Yes, she realized the need. But two months is the earliest clinic appointment she
can offer. No, she was sorry, but she couldn't guarantee that Dr. Long
himself would do the examination. There was a group of very good
physicians at the Pain Clinic.

Sorry. Two months was the soonest.

Fran tuned the conversation out. She frowned once more at the calendar, closed it, and returned to her typing.

On the morning of the twelfth, as on all mornings, one of the first
things she did was open the calendar, and the first thing she saw was
her notation about the alert.

By then Dr. Murray was already standing in front of the X-ray
board in the operating room. Behind him Joe Trott lay, heavily
sedated, on the steel table.

A resident stopped to stand for a moment beside Dr. Murray, looking at the scans.

Big, huh?

Yeah.

College student.

The resident studied the scans.

Wow.

In the past week Dr. Murray and Dr. Long had spent considerable
time poring over the films. Ordinarily Dr. Murray would handle a
case like this himself, but this one . . . it was interesting enough that
Dr. Long would want to see it and dangerous enough for Dr. Murray
to want him to.

Dr. Murray had decided, and Dr. Long had agreed, that there were
two major possibilities and a smattering of minor ones.

According to all the radiology textbooks, Joe Trott's tumor should
be a meningioma, a noncancerous growth that begins in the meninges,
the layers of membrane that protect the brain and its parts. A meningioma was difficult to recognize on a CAT scan, but it was easy to
identify when you saw it. It had a characteristic brown color.

Until then, the diagnosis was tricky.

Meningiomas had the peculiar ability to make blood vessels grow toward them. As a result, they showed up on an angiogram as a dense tangle of arteries and veins.

An angiogram involves injecting a contrast medium into the blood to outline the vessels of the brain. Like all tumor patients, Joe Trott had one. In fact, he had several. To look at the tangle of vessels on the resulting films, his tumor was a meningioma.

That would be good for Joe, since meningiomas were usually soft and were relatively easy to extract. They weren't cancerous but, unfortunately, meningiomas often recurred in ten years or so.

It could also be an off-the-wall cancer, one of the quick and vicious ones, a sarcoma, perhaps, or an angioblastoma. Those were wild cards that had to be considered.

But neither of the surgeons thought the tumor was one of those. And despite the vessels, they didn't think it was a meningioma.

Significantly, one of Joe's first symptoms was a hearing loss, and later he heard . . . it wasn't the classic ringing. It was more like a mosquito buzzing in his ear, a mosquito that was always with him but wasn't there. Whatever he heard, it was a phony noise.

There was another sort of tumor that occasionally developed dense vasculature. It arose from the eighth cranial nerve, otherwise known as the acoustic nerve, the nerve that attaches the ear to the brain.

Along with the twenty-two other nerves that control the lips, tongue, face and head muscles, the two acoustic nerves lie in the bottom of the posterior fossa, beneath the lizard brain.

It was interesting, if you were a student and attracted to Great Questions. It was interesting that a handshake was relayed through channels, down through the spinal cord. A smile came directly from the lizard brain.

But as Dr. Murray stood in front of Joe Trott's CAT scans, he thought nothing of that. He thought of anatomy, and structure, and cell types.

One reason Dr. Long had wooed Dr. Murray to the Hopkins was the junior surgeon's postdoctoral work in tumor immunology. That, and the fact that Dr. Murray had studied neurosurgery under the same demanding surgeon who had trained Dr. Long. The combination of clinical and laboratory experience gave Dr. Murray a valuable dual viewpoint. He examined Joe's CAT scans from the twin perspectives of scientist and surgeon.

Despite the blood vessels, Joe's problem was probably an acoustic tumor—an acoustic neurinoma to be more accurate, a giant acoustic neurinoma to be absolutely precise. On rare occasions, they too attracted blood vessels.

They weren't brown. They were yellow.

From Joe Trott's point of view, the possibility contained both good and bad news. The good news was that acoustic tumors, if carefully removed, didn't grow back.

If you could get them out.

A giant meningioma in the posterior fossa wasn't a piece of cake, by any means. Dr. Murray wouldn't like to try one anywhere but in a large teaching hospital, where he had plenty of equipment, a good microscope and an experienced team.

You had to expose the tumor, cut into it and remove it from the inside first. If you did it right, it collapsed on you. Then you could tease it away from the brain stem and strip it off the basilar artery.

It wasn't as though a giant meningioma was easy. It was not. But a giant acoustic neurinoma was even worse. The procedure was roughly the same, until it came time to strip its membrane off the brain stem and basilar artery. The membrane of an acoustic neurinoma stuck tight to everything.

The trick was to find a layer where the bond was weak, the way the bond is weak between an orange and its skin, or an old egg and its shell. Surgeons called that a plane, and if you could find a plane you could peel, not pull. If you can find a plane an acoustic tumor can be removed.

If, in the process of removing an acoustic tumor, you left one tiny bit of abnormal tissue, the whole damned thing grew back, and it was mixed with scar tissue. Since scar tissue stuck to everything, too, and since it was almost indistinguishable from tumor, a regrown acoustic neurinoma was almost impossible to remove.

If it was a neurinoma, Dr. Murray had decided, he'd call Dr. Long. He would want Dr. Long to be involved in any neurinoma that size.

Seven stories above Dr. Murray's operating room, Dr. Long entered his office, removed his topcoat and hung it up. Then he slipped on a fresh white laboratory jacket. Absently, he removed an old-fashioned hatpin from yesterday's jacket and pushed it through his clean, starched lapel.

Fran Crow stuck her head through the door. You're on alert today. The Trott case, yes sir. Dr. Murray's in the OR now. In the meantime the chief of neurosurgery had letters to sign, patients to examine, residents to interview and visitors to see.

Downstairs, in the operating room, Dr. Murray stood over Joe Trott. The young man's hand moved, awkwardly, in recognition.

We're all set, Joe.

The anesthesiologist leaned close over the patient's face. "You're going to feel sleepy now." A few seconds later Joe was unconscious. The anesthesiologist inserted a plastic tube down his patient's windpipe.

The operating room was crowded with personnel, checking electronics equipment, laying out tools, and some just watching. Near the table, a nurse and a technician worked to assemble a Mayfield clamp. The clamp was a large, gangly apparatus of jointed steel. The nurse held it steady in the proper position while the technician tightened the bolts to stiffen the joints.

At the top of the clamp was a set of sharp pincers, about the size of a set of heavy-duty ice tongs. The operating room lights glinted harshly from its honed tips.

The heart monitor beeped steadily, seventy beats a minute, perfect.

Upstairs, in his office, Dr. Long sorted through a pile of pink telephone-message forms, dividing them into two stacks. When he finished he took the smaller stack out to Fran and Pat. They picked up their telephones to find the people Dr. Long wanted to talk to.

While he waited, Dr. Long sat at his desk and dictated letters to the remaining callers. As the secretaries connected him with various people, he put the dictaphone aside.

Yes, he would present a paper at an upcoming meeting.

No, he didn't do that kind of back surgery any more, but he knew the name of a fine neurosurgeon in the community.

That sounds interesting. Make an appointment for clinic . . .

A blank television monitor sat nearby, ready in case Dr. Murray wanted an instant consultation. At the touch of a switch, Dr. Long's monitor could echo the picture on the screen downstairs.

In his office, Dr. Long was surrounded by organized clutter. Diplomas, certificates and other trophies of academic victories decorated the walls. X-ray films hung, lopsided, on a darkened display board, the outlines of a skull indistinct without backlighting. Stacks of slides and publications covered the coffee table.

There was no coffee pot. Coffee would make his hands shake.

As the Harvey Cushing Professor of Neurosurgery and chief of the department, Dr. Long rated a corner office. Picture windows on two walls let in the gray March sunlight. Below and to the north, thousands of row houses dominated the gentle hills of Baltimore. The dark smoke rising from the chimneys was almost instantly whipped away by the wind.

Downstairs, the residents had shaved Joe Trott's scalp and attached the Mayfield clamp to the table. Ten hands lifted Joe to a sitting position. The clamp bit through his scalp and gouged into the bone. Using a square of gauze, a resident wiped away the trickles of blood.

With Dr. Murray giving commands, the team readjusted the boy's position, loosening and retightening the bolts.

The tilt of the head should be more, yes, that way. The ear should be about right there. No. No, on second thought, tilted more to the left. Yes. There. Right.

The team gave the bolts one more turn for good measure and cautiously stepped back.

Half-propped against the raised back of the table, half-hanging from the Mayfield clamp, Joe sat in a slumped-forward position, chin tucked in. He could have been dozing in class.

Thoughtfully, Dr. Murray walked outside to the scrub sink.

He would be approaching the tumor through the back of the head. With the neck muscles stripped away he could reach the underside of the skull, where the bone is thin and can be bitten away with long-handled nippers.

First, however, Dr. Murray would have to deal with the pressure in the boy's head, and with the time-bomb situation that had prompted the neurosurgeon to insist on the wheelchair.

Because the tumor had blocked the flow of spinal fluid out of the brain, the pressure had risen. As high as it was now, if he cut a hole in the skull the pressure would probably send the brain matter oozing out at him, like warm gray toothpaste out of a burst tube.

By the time he had scrubbed, gowned and gloved, two assistants had already begun preparing to reduce the pressure. Now, with Dr. Murray watching, they used a pneumatic drill to make a very small hole in the top of Joe's head. Then they pushed a fine, hollow needle down into the brain, toward one of the big main ventricles.

When the probe pierced the ventricle wall, clear fluid fountained out and rained on their sterile gowns. As the pressure subsided inside the skull, the fountain died to a dribble.

The spinal fluid was clear, which was reassuring. Pressure can sometimes cause hemorrhage inside the brain but, were that the case, the fluid would have been pink.

The residents attached the drain to a piece of plastic tubing and put a bandage over the hole. Then they moved around to the back of the patient and set about rearranging their equipment.

Dr. Murray traced his finger along the back of Joe's head, not quite touching the flesh. The resident's scalpel cut deep and, for an instant, the raw flesh was white. Then the incision filled with blood.

The surgical march into the brain is ancient, almost as ancient as man. Archaeologists have found half-fossilized skulls bearing what are certainly surgical holes. The holes were scraped, carefully. Even then, whoever did it knew he had to be careful, very careful, while working around the brain.

Why did they do it? Nobody knows. Perhaps they were letting the demons out, or the gods in. In the South Pacific, trephining, as it's called, was apparently a rite of manhood.

Whatever the reason, they did it, and they did it well. Many of the skulls have bone-scar tissue around the raw edges of the hole, indicating that the patient/victim lived for some time following the trephining.

Other skulls show signs of fulminating bone infection, indicating that the trephinee lived for a while and then died of infection. Then as now neurosurgery was a high-risk proposition.

On the other hand, the fact that many people recovered tells neurosurgeons that the trephiners, whoever they were, weren't really brain surgeons. They may have gone through the skull, but they didn't open the dura. If they had opened the dura under nonsterile conditions, the brain itself would have become infected and turned to liquid.

Working directly behind Joe Trott's head, Dr. Murray and his resident cut around a large flap of tissue. When they had finished, the incision began behind Joe's left ear, arched upward toward the crown of his head, and fell back down to the neck. The flap itself was about the size of Dr. Murray's hand.

The two worked quickly to stanch the bleeding. The flesh of the head is rich with blood vessels. You can bleed to death from a scalp wound.

Nobody knows how the ancient trephiners solved the problem. With hot coals, maybe. Modern surgeons are more ingenious.

"Scalp clips," Dr. Murray said.

The nurse laid a long, pliers-like instrument in his hand. An attachment on its tip held what surgeons call a barrel clip, a length of hard plastic tubing split lengthwise. The instrument held the slit open until the scalp's cut edge was inside the jaws. Then it snapped shut, squeezing off the blood flow.

The clip forceps clattered back onto the scrub nurse's table and she laid another pair in the surgeon's gloved hand. Then another, and another.

When the incision was finished and the bleeding stopped, Joe looked as though he had two lines of small hair curlers running upward from his left ear and falling down the midline of his skull.

The heart monitor beeped steadily.

The incision outlined Joe's neck muscle where it attached to the skull. The resident ran a chisel between flesh and bone, severing the union. While he scraped, a junior resident found the bleeders with the bipolars and burned them shut.

There is a ritual. Catch the bleeder. Burn it. Wipe the cut end of the muscle with a gauze sponge. Examine the burned bleeder. If it still oozes blood, zap it again.

Beneath the large outer muscle there are seven other muscles. Patiently, the residents cut each away from the skull with the chisel.

Dr. Murray stood, watching the residents work. He had done such chores, once, but as a teacher he now did them only rarely. It would be unfair.

With the law as tight as it is today, you can't often let your residents operate on the brain itself. But you have to let them do all they can. They can do approaches. And retreats. Open and close. Open and close. A resident might open and close hundreds of heads before ever touching a living human brain.

The chisel grated against the bone as the muscle and underlying tissue were scraped away. Dr. Murray watched, patiently.

Nearby, a burly male nurse tinkered with a large black nitrogen bottle on a moving cart. He freed the cart and carefully rolled it toward the operating table. The scrub nurse laid out a long, pressurized tube that had been gas-sterilized. She handed one end of the tube to the man, being careful not to touch him and contaminate her gloves.

The scrub nurse's end of the hose was still sterile. She plugged it into a large metal tool that looked very much like a mechanic's impact wrench.

Testing, she said, and pulled the trigger.

Zhoop. Zhoop. Zhooooooooooooooooo.

It took several minutes for the residents to scrape the back of the skull clean and identify the anatomical landmarks. The area of interest was up under the back of the skull, where the spine attaches to it. That area is usually well protected by the bulging neck muscles. Nature, always frugal, made the bone thinner there.

The senior resident studied the exposed bone. Finally, without prompting, he put a gloved fingertip on the ivory bone.

Dr. Murray nodded, pleased.

Yes. Right there.

"Craniotome," the resident said, and the nurse laid the power drill in his hand. He held it for a moment while she carefully arranged the trailing gas hose so it wouldn't get in the way.

When she was satisfied, the resident pressed the bit against the bone. Zhoooooooooooooo . . .

Bone filings curled up around the hole.

. . . ooooooooooooooooooooooooooooooooop.

A pressure sensor in the bit shut the drill off the instant it encountered the soft dura. The resident withdrew the craniotome and handed it back to the scrub nurse. The bone was about three sixteenths of an inch thick, and the hole was the size of a dime. Its raw sides oozed blood.

Bone wax, please.

The scrub nurse placed a tiny ball of soft wax on the resident's index finger, and he pressed it into the raw bone. The oozing stopped immediately.

At the bottom of the hole, the dura mater shined a dull gray.

The residents moved on, without hesitation.

"Rongeur, please."

The small, bone-biting pliers fitted perfectly into the resident's palm.

The bone need not be replaced, not down here, under so many protective muscles. It was easier, and therefore safer, to bite it away.

Again and again, the instrument crunched down. The resident pulled the bone fragments free with a practiced flip of his wrist, keeping the motion always out, away from the brain.

When a two-inch hole in the bone had been cleared, Dr. Murray used his fingertips to carefully palpate the dura, and the brain behind it.

Fine. There didn't seem to be too much pressure.

The heart monitor beeped regularly.

A tiny hook lifted the dura clear of the brain, and a scalpel parted it. Below, the brightly striped convolutions of the cerebellum glistened in the surgical spotlight.

The brain is far more like a computer network than a single computer, and each of its subsystems evolved in an individual direction. The part of the brain that now blocked Dr. Murray's advance was the left hemisphere of the cerebellum, the body's automatic pilot.

The cerebellum sits in the lower rear of the brain, a Chinaman's knot just behind the brain stem. It allows its owner to make complex, co-ordinated movements without thinking about it. When Joe wanted to move his right hand the cerebellum told the necessary muscles to tighten. It gave him the ability to walk, drive or scratch his back without conscious effort.

Fortunately, the cerebellum is somewhat less critical than other parts of the brain. Nature's design allowed for a little extra core space, so Dr. Murray, if he's cautious, can push aside the cerebellum. Not push exactly, of course, but move it, anyway. Cells will die, but Joe won't be particularly affected.

For that matter, it's even possible to cut away a third of the cerebellum. The worst that would happen would be that it would take Joe a millisecond longer to slap a mosquito.

Still, no procedure was without risk. And cutting it away might take Dr. Murray a bit too close to the anterior inferior cerebellar artery.

The anterior inferior cerebellar artery arises from the big basilar artery and runs up along the undersurface of the cerebellum, where it divides into smaller vessels. Most of those vessels feed the cerebellum, and are of minor note.

But a few very small branches, microscopic ones almost, dive into the adjacent brain stem and supply the reticular formation. The reticular formation was not forgiving at all.

If Dr. Murray inadvertently touched one of those tiny vessels, it might rupture. A half inch away, some small clump of gray neurons would die, a signal would cease, and something would happen. When it did, the surgeon sometimes didn't even know about it. He would do the rest of the operation perfectly, and send the patient out into the recovery room to wake up. Only he never would. The medical students would come around and look at him, and speculate about what was missing.

Every brain surgeon learned about the anterior inferior cerebellar artery in neuroanatomy class. Experience in the operating room elevated the knowledge to fear.

The anterior inferior cerebellar artery wasn't just a piece of anatomical geography. It wasn't like an artery that fed the big toe, or a centimeter of the gut. It ran right into the center of the universe. It waited there, tiny in proportion to its danger, hiding, patient, malevolent, a paw of the . . . the . . . the Something.

It wasn't the "anterior inferior cerebellar artery" to Dr. Murray.

It was the *aye-ka*.

Anterior Inferior Cerebellar Artery. AICA.

Spoken sharply, *aye-ka*. Like an ancient Nile god of the night, *aye-ka*.

Gently, tentatively, Dr. Murray lifted the bottom of the cerebellum. He could cut, but he'd rather lift. If he cut, he might disturb the aye-ka.

Retracting the cerebellum, as the moving-back process is called, is a subject of absorbing interest to brain surgeons. There are papers written on it, scholarly catfights over how best to do it, and a variety of gadgets, called cerebellar retractors, to make it easier.

When a neurosurgeon pushes his way beneath a sac of brain tissue, he enters a microscopic tunnel in which the throbbing walls and ceilings threaten, moment by moment, to cave in. All that prevents disaster are the two thin, transparent inner membranes of the meninges.

The arachnoid is the outermost, and it wraps the major inner structures of the brain, like the cerebellum. Beneath that the pia, a final membrane, follows the folds of brain as they dip in and then reappear again, convolution after convolution.

The pia is the innermost and most delicate of the membranes, and behind it lies the runny gray goo that thinks. The trick is to somehow pry that sac of goo back without rupturing the pia. Only a retractor makes that possible.

The cerebellar retractor favored by Dr. Murray is a spindly thing with jutting arms and metal tentacles that can be locked into place with the turn of a handscrew. Each tentacle holds a long, smooth, flat, easily bent piece of metal. Carefully, Dr. Murray used the pieces of metal to push the cerebellum aside.

Of course, not pushing. Not really. You get under it, not lifting, more encouraging, wishing it up . . .

Once you've got it where you want it, and if the pia hasn't ripped, you tighten the screw and lock it in place. Then, behind the lenses of the microscope, you go in. Above you, the ceiling pulses and heaves, straining against the thin membranes.

Carefully, carefully, Dr. Murray bent the retractors. Every touch left a red bruise on the surface of the cerebellum.

The work totally absorbed the neurosurgeon and his assistants. The scrub nurse handed them tools, saying nothing. The anesthesiologist watched the dials jump back and forth, back and forth, back and forth, with Joe's every breath.

Finally the cerebellum was high enough that Dr. Murray could see behind and beyond, into the brain.

He adjusted the light and peered in.

A yellowish, slick surface glittered wetly back at him.

Yellow.

Yellow, not brown.

So much for the meningioma.

Dr. Long would want to see this.

CHAPTER
TEN

UPSTAIRS, IN HIS OFFICE, DR. LONG POPPED THE MICROCASSETTE OUT OF his dictaphone. He stood, stretched, and adjusted his white lab coat. His fingers were disproportionately small, compared to the surgeon's slightly stocky body. A small frown crossed his normally placid features. There were many more letters to dictate, but it was time for pain rounds. At least he got some of the correspondence out of the way.

Again this weekend he'd have to take his dictaphone home with him to catch up. Usually he had to take it with him on vacation, too. When that happened, he mailed Fran the cassettes.

Personally he'd rather spend more of his time in the operating rooms, or the laboratories. But the honor of the Harvey Cushing Chair in Neurosurgery was accompanied by a variety of administrative responsibilities. One of those was answering a steady flood of mail from people who were far, far too important to ignore.

Tossing the cassette thoughtfully in his hand, he walked to the doorway of his office. Pain rounds was another of his obligations that he didn't always relish, but that wasn't something he could blame on Harvey Cushing and Walter Dandy. That one he'd brought on himself.

Dr. Long stopped in the doorway, next to Fran's desk. His administrative secretary was on the telephone with somebody who rated the yes-sir-no-sir treatment.

Yes sir, Dr. Murray, hold on, he's right here. Fran handed the receiver to Dr. Long.

The operating room speakerphone added a slight echo to Dr. Murray's voice. They were definitely dealing with an acoustic tumor, Dr. Murray said, though he'd send a bit to pathology for the record. Did Dr. Long want to come down now?

Dr. Long hesitated. His preference was to go to the operating room, but conscience said otherwise. He really should attend pain rounds.

After a moment of discussion it was agreed that Dr. Long would see to the pain patients and that Dr. Murray would forge ahead. The junior surgeon could cut into the tumor and gut, or debulk, it. Dr. Long would get to the operating room later on, and take over in time to peel it from the basilar artery and the brain stem. That would be the scary part, anyway. Maybe, he hoped, the thing wouldn't be stuck too tightly.

Dr. Long handed the telephone back to Fran, and then tossed her the cassette. Dr. Murray might have to reach him quickly.

"Yes, sir," Fran said. In her mind, the nature of the alert changed. Now it was Red Alert.

Downstairs in the operating room, Dr. Murray walked away from the speakerphone back to his patient. As the operating room team draped the microscope in clear, sterile plastic, he stood looking at the exposed brain. The retraction of the cerebellum had created a long crevice. At its bottom, the yellow tumor glistened ominously.

Maybe, just maybe, it wouldn't be stuck too tightly.

He stepped forward to lend a hand as the crew swung the instrument around, carefully, carefully . . . just . . . right . . . there.

Lights off.

The bulbs in the spotlights glowed briefly and then the room was dark. The scrub nurse blinked, her pupils expanding.

Dr. Murray pressed his eyes against the microscope, adjusting the focus and the tiny headlight.

The microscope thrust him up close, into the brain. Overhead, the cerebellum strained downward against the stretched arachnoid and pia membranes, held away only by the retractors. The yellow tumor appeared on the television monitor.

First, the aye-ka.

Dr. Murray wanted to see it with his own two eyes, visualize it, as neurosurgeons say, know exactly where it was, without question, without doubt. Only in that way could he be certain not to touch it accidentally.

Dr. Murray quickly visualized the aye-ka, and pointed it out to his assistant at the side 'scope. See? Right there. The assistant frowned into the microscope, straining. Then he relaxed. Sure. There. Right there.

Partly concealed in a cocoon of white connective fibers, it pulsated threateningly. Both surgeons stared at it, fixing its position in their minds. They would be putting instruments into the hole and taking them out. They'd be sucking away the tumor. There would be minor detours, and bleeders, and puzzles to unravel, and maybe even a white-faced panic or two.

But never for a moment, not for an instant, would either surgeon forget exactly where his instrument was in relation to the aye-ka.

Upstairs, Dr. Long had arranged for the Red Alert, given Fran the telephone number, and was ready to be off. If it hadn't been his month to conduct pain rounds . . . but he *had* to go sometime, after all.

Because Johns Hopkins was the birthplace of neurosurgery, Dr. Long naturally got calls from kings and presidents. Interesting patients were referred to him because, after all, they were tough cases, and the Hopkins was good at handling tough cases. Dr. Long loved the challenges that Harvey Cushing's ghost brought him.

But the patients who came to the Pain Clinic from all over the world didn't, as a rule, have the vaguest idea who Harvey Cushing was. They came because they had heard of Dr. Long. They had waited months for an appointment.

In the generality of medical practice, it was a good thing, a very good thing, to have a waiting room full of people. But in Dr. Long's case, the waiting room, if he let it, would be full of people who were addicted to pain, and . . .

He had known better, really. And he hadn't done it on purpose. But he had been young, and bright, and out to do good for the world.

Not that he was the flighty sort who would sit around endlessly in the campus tavern consuming gallons of draft beer and pontificating on the soul. Nothing like that at all. His early studies had been in no-nonsense physics, and he had wanted to use science, hard science, to help people.

He had gravitated directly to the nuts-and-bolts aspect of the brain, to the microscopic circuitry, which was where the action was. If he had wanted to waste his time on great truths, he would have chosen a less tangible specialty, like psychology.

As his residency ended, Dr. Long accepted a position as a neurosurgeon at the University of Minnesota Hospital. That was in the early 1960s, and while he had finally earned the right to wear the hatpin in his lapel, he still wasn't finished paying dues.

It was his job, as junior man, to take care of the depressing patients that his seniors preferred to avoid. One of the things most neurosurgeons would prefer to avoid was, and still is, pain patients.

Not that pain patients couldn't be rewarding. When young Dr. Long severed the pain pathways in a cancer victim, he made it possible for that person to die in peace. When he performed an operation on a man's back and the man returned to work, well, that made it a good day.

But if those were typical pain cases, professors of neurosurgery wouldn't slough them off onto their assistants. In practice, pain surgery usually made you feel inadequate and guilty.

Most of the time, no matter how much experience you had, no matter where you learned your trade, or how perfectly you operated—something went wrong. The pain, if it subsided at all, soon returned in full, brutal force. Sometimes it was even worse than before. And the patient, who had once trusted the surgeon, now looked at him with tortured, accusing eyes.

The tradition of neurosurgery holds that it was a good thing for junior neurosurgeons to do pain cases. Junior neurosurgeons, having survived their residencies, sometimes tended to swagger and think highly of themselves. Pain patients kept them humble.

But it was expected that the junior neurosurgeon would take the punishment only until an even younger neurosurgeon joined the staff. The younger man, then, would become the institution's pain expert.

But young Donlin Long was touched by the suffering people who came to him. Most of them had had several back operations already, and had been doctor-shopping all over the country. He tested them and studied them, and became convinced they weren't faking it. They were in pain, all right, and it was ruining their lives.

To make it even more compelling, most of the patients were women, and they all too frequently reminded a young neurosurgeon of his mother, sister, or wife. They were desperate, they begged for help.

What strange, undiscovered disease made them suffer so? Why, when he operated on them, and operated perfectly, did their pain disappear . . . and then come back? What *was* pain, anyway?

So young Donlin Long didn't bide his time and await the arrival of an even greener neurosurgeon. The next time a junior man arrived on the staff, he was spared the ordeal. He didn't get the pain cases, because by then Donlin Long wanted to keep them.

There was something important there. Very important. He was certain of it. It had to do, somehow, with the nature of pain. Pain was a stimulus that traveled up the nerves, into the spinal cord and then to the brain. There, circuits opened and closed, neurons pumped chemicals at one another, and pain was produced. Pain happened in the brain, not the mashed finger or the broken leg.

With the pain patients, somewhere along the line, the circuits must have been shorted out or something. Perhaps the nerves sent erroneous messages, or something that was attached to something became, for some reason, attached instead to something else.

Dr. Long studied the origins and mechanisms of pain, mapping its paths up the nerve to the nerve root, next to the spinal cord, and from there to the cord itself. The path led him, finally, to a subsystem of the lizard brain called the thalamus.

By that time scientists already knew the thalamus was where pain happened. Not in the aching back, but in the brain. That was why, they theorized, hypnotism could defuse dental pain, and why a person in a religious trance could turn off some switch in his head and walk across hot coals.

The people young Dr. Long saw were not truly representative. Usually, a neurosurgeon in the suburbs was able to trace the pain to a pinched nerve in the back or neck, and then, as a matter of routine, he fixed it. In fact, back and neck operations are the most common operations in neurosurgery.

Dr. Long's patients had already been that route. By the time they came to Dr. Long they might have been that route several times. There was often so much scar tissue around their spinal cords that the young neurosurgeon despaired of ever finding out what was wrong.

Examining such patients, Dr. Long was forced to confront the fact that some of his colleagues were not, how could he put it, weren't exactly, well . . . some of the old operations he saw made him shudder. A lot of the operations had been conceived on a faulty knowledge of anatomy and physiology; many had been done without very good follow-up of the results. Maybe some of the pain had actually been caused by the first neurosurgeon.

Perhaps there had never been anything wrong with the back, in the first place. Perhaps there had been no pinched nerve at all. Perhaps the nerve pathways, or the pain centers in the thalamus itself, were somehow damaged. Perhaps a circuit had shorted, or a chemical thermostat had malfunctioned. Perhaps, then, the thalamus heard pain signals that weren't there.

That would explain a lot. No back or neck operation would cure such pain. Perhaps, if that were the case, Dr. Long could somehow override the pain circuits . . . perhaps with an electrode in the brain. After all, electrodes could override circuits in cats and even, one scientist had shown, in angry bulls.

That was one of the classics of bioscience. A fellow by the name of Delgado had started by implanting electrodes in the emotional centers of usually aggressive dominant monkeys. With a tingle of electricity in the right place, he discovered, he could make the monkeys temporarily meek. With a few more, he could make their personalities change permanently.

But his most famous demonstration involved a fighting bull in his homeland, Spain. Delgado implanted an electrode in the pleasure center of the bull's brain, then attached the electrode to a tiny radio receiver on the outside of the animal's head.

When the animal had recovered, the scientist walked into a bullring with it, armed only with a small radio transmitter. Hundreds of spectators watched.

The bull snorted, pawed the ground, bellowed in rage, and charged.

The scientist pushed the button on his transmitter.

Surprise flickered through the bull's brain, followed by pleasure.

Then a half ton of fighting bull skidded to a stop in a cloud of dust and a rising wind of love, love, sweet love for the nice man with the pretty box.

Could Donlin Long do that for people in pain?

Dr. Long reviewed the scientific literature on the subject. Only a few neurosurgeons had experimented with pain-killing electrodes.

First in cats and later in humans, he experimented with electrodes surgically implanted into specific areas of the brain and spinal cord. He was elated when he found that, in many instances, a mild electric current applied to nerve roots along the spinal cord could indeed block the pain signals.

Later, he discovered that electrodes carefully placed in the patient's brain could produce a similar result. To keep the pain blocked, however, the electrode had to remain in place in the brain, and electricity had to be kept flowing through it at a measured rate. As a general practice, the risk of infection made leaving the electrodes in too dangerous.

Throughout the early experiments, Dr. Long urged his patients to describe what they felt when they turned on the electricity. The patients groped for words. One of the most frequent observations was that it felt like a sort of "tingling" that covered the pain. The pain was still there . . . but it didn't hurt.

The tingling feeling suggested a solution to the infection problem. What if, instead of using an electrode in the brain, he sent the tingling sensation up the brain's natural electrodes, the nerves? Would a tingle of electricity, applied to the nerves through the skin, work as well to kill the pain?

The answer was yes.

Dr. Long teamed up with bioengineers to develop a battery-powered tingler. Experimentation in the clinic determined precisely where on the body the electrodes should be attached, and how much electricity was needed to kill the pain. Then the patients could go home.

The miniaturized tingler was no problem at all. It was only about the size of a small transistor radio, and it could be worn on the belt. If the patient were sensitive, he could easily conceal it in a pocket or under his clothing.

And then, with many of the patients, Donlin Long ran into the same brick wall as had his predecessors. The pain went away, all right. But it came back.

Dr. Long had seen the same phenomenon with the spinal cord implants, and had puzzled over it at some length without finding any answers. Now the same thing was happening with the skin-stimulators. Why?

He checked and rechecked the equipment. Everything would be working perfectly, except that nothing worked at all. And the women looked at him with sad, accusing eyes.

What was he doing wrong?

In the eyes of the public, nothing.

The pain work had an immediate appeal to the press, and stories about it moved on the wire services. Dr. Long, at the University of Minnesota, was doing something for victims of chronic pain, for people who had been turned away by doctor after doctor.

As Dr. Long was about to discover, many chronic pain patients had little to do besides hurt, complain, clip newspaper stories, write letters, and make telephone calls.

Many of those telephone calls went to local newspapers, and medical writers discovered that chronic pain patients made interesting and moving feature stories. Those stories generated still more telephone calls and very quickly, just as Dr. Long was beginning to get that chilly feeling that something was wrong, very wrong . . . he became famous.

There were a lot of chronic pain patients, a whole lot of them. Dr. Long had never dreamed how many.

He tried to help as many as he could with implanted electrodes, or if possible the tingler, and the pain would go away.

In some, it didn't come back. But for far too many, it did. Why?

As the months passed, Dr. Long noticed an odd distinction between the patients who got better and the ones who didn't. The ones who got better were the sensitive ones—the ones who hid the tingler under their clothes. The ones whose pain recurred were usually those who wore it on the outside.

Now what on earth did *that* mean?

It sounded more like a question in psychology than one in neurosurgery, but Dr. Long was desperate, and he focused his powers of scientific observation on his patients' behavior. The answer, once he found it, seemed fiendishly simple.

Dr. Long didn't need to know much psychology to conclude that the patients who concealed the tingler did so because they were ashamed of being abnormal.

But to the others, the tingler was a visible badge of suffering. Far from being ashamed, they were proud. They were eager to talk about it to friends and co-workers, to recount the agony they'd suffered, and how they had been brushed aside by one doctor after another, and how finally this one man, this wonderful Dr. Long . . .

If the listener was at all sympathetic, he listened a long time. And, after a few months, or a year, when the novelty of the gizmo wore off, and the conversational possibilities were exhausted, the pain returned.

It was real pain, too, Dr. Long was convinced. It had been real before, as well. He had blocked the circuits, and it had subsided, but then . . .

Had the circuits rewired themselves, and routed the ghost pain signals around the tingler's block? Why would the brain do that?

Dr. Long started asking questions about the patients' home lives, about their husbands, and children, and about their relationships with their mothers. He was dumbfounded by their answers, and the motives he saw behind them.

The pain came back when the patient was lonely. Pain brought sympathy. Pain was an excuse for every guilty imperfection. Pain made your family and friends take you seriously. Pain made you special. It even got you fussed over by a big-shot doctor.

The primitive lizard brain, where the pain centers are, harkens back to a time long before the coal forests, and the last ice age, and the appearance of man. The lizard brain works silently, far beneath the range of consciousness. It makes its judgement and it moves, unseen and unfelt. It rewires the brain to suit its most basic purposes.

But pain? Pain is awful. Why would the lizard want to hurt?

The answer didn't come from neurosurgery, it came from poetry, and music, and the conversations in beer halls.

Pain is terrible. Only one thing is worse: loneliness.

Dr. Long, while innocently working in the area of wiring diagrams, had broken through to the psyche. He couldn't cure them because they wouldn't let him. They didn't dare. They *needed* their pain.

Dr. Long reported in the scientific journals that there were two types of pain, physical and psychological. Pain caused by physical problems—slipped discs pressing on nerve roots, for instance—could often be surgically corrected. But when dealing with the other kind of pain, the psychologically-induced pain, the surgeon had to be very careful lest the doctor-patient relationship actually keep the pain alive. To identify such patients and treat them, the neurosurgeon needed to collaborate with a psychiatrist.

Above all, the surgeon should not let the patients perceive that pain could earn them the sympathetic attention of a doctor.

But for Dr. Long, it was too late. Thanks to the newspaper articles and the free endorsements from his big-mouthed patients, he was a marked man. They came to him, now, by the thousands.

He got begging letters, written in painful, cramped penmanship, that related heart-wrenching stories of agony, of pain-wracked lives, stories guaranteed to strike guilt and obligation into a neurosurgeon's soul.

Please, doctor. Nobody else will help me!

The calls were worse. There was a whine to the voices, a desperation to the words, that made Dr. Long want to help, but usually he could do nothing but examine them and recommend a psychiatrist. Then they would look at him with pitiful eyes, forgiving him perhaps for this last offense to their anguished psyches. But he could do nothing, he'd say.

It was a weak argument, because often they didn't really expect him to do anything, except listen. And he didn't *want* to be a psychologist.

He had other things to do, tumor patients to save, cancer patients with real pain to ease, crippled people with back problems he could really fix. He didn't have time to listen, but he couldn't stop them from calling. The pleas were full of immediacy.

The neurosurgical wards were full of people with terrible diseases, with malformations and tumors, with aneurysms and severed nerves, and each case was, in its own way, urgent.

But none of them, not even glioblastoma multiforme, was as urgent as pain. Glioblastoma multiforme kills tomorrow, not today. Pain is today, this hour, right now.

To survive the stresses of neurosurgery, every surgeon develops a hobby, a coping mechanism, that allows for escape. Michael Salcman fled into the world of art collecting and scuba diving. Tom Ducker sailed. Donlin Long walked in his garden, and watered, and spread leaf mold, and pruned trees, and made things grow.

His garden was a private world to him, a happy reminder of childhood summers on his grandparents' farm in Missouri. It was almost, but not quite, as good as bass fishing back home in Missouri. Most of all it was peace inviolate.

Well, almost inviolate.

The day came, as his fame grew, that even his garden could not protect him.

It was a Saturday, and there was a fruit tree that needed trimming. A branch near the top was rubbing against another branch, and it had to come down. It was a tricky chore, but a pleasant one. A tree never, ever, screams.

The neurosurgeon in him was far away, the gardener was in the ascendancy, and he whistled as he gathered together the necessary equipment. He carefully propped the ladder in the tree, took the chain saw in hand, and climbed into the foliage. Once there he balanced himself carefully and pulled the starter on the chain saw. It roared immediately to life, and he gunned it a couple of times, to warm it up. Then he reached out and prepared to press its flashing teeth against the wood.

And the ladder shook.

Reacting instantly, the neurosurgeon grabbed a branch with his free hand, steadying himself. The ladder shook again.

Peering down through the leaves, he saw a stranger leaning on the ladder and looking up at him.

The ladder rocked again.

Dr. Long held the chain saw away from his body. A neurosurgeon with fewer than ten intact fingers wouldn't be much good for anything but giving lectures.

Doc, the man said, *you gotta help me.*

Donlin Long clung to the branch. There was no way to turn off the chain saw without letting go of the branch.

Please, Doc.

The chain saw!

Please, Doc.

The ladder!

Doctor, it's been terrible . . .

It was the last straw. Or, if not the last straw, a straw very near the last. Something had to be done.

Dr. Long was far too famous to back out now, and he thought he could help some of the people with psychiatric pain. He needed to separate them from patients who really needed surgery, and get them into a psychiatric clinic. Or somewhere. Certainly not in his garden.

It was no accident that Dr. Long's Pain Center was located three buildings and fourteen floors away from the departmental offices. The patients didn't come to see Dr. Long; he went to see them.

In that fashion, and in others, he sought diligently to limit pain patients to no more than twenty-five percent of his practice.

The irony was made all the more acute by the fact that Dr. Long's place in the medical history books had nothing at all to do with pain. It had to do instead with his pioneering research into steroid therapy, and the swelling of the brain.

The first big advance in brain surgery had come at the turn of the century, when young Harvey Cushing had ignored the sage advice of his seniors and began cutting into the brain. The second major advance came in the 1950s and '60s, with the introduction of the operating microscope.

Then, for a time, the development of neurosurgery seemed blocked by the brain's tendency to bruise at the slightest touch, and for the bruised neurons to swell. If the surgeon tried to do very much, something happened.

The patient didn't die on the table. He woke up after the surgery, and seemed fine. But a few hours later, as his brain swelled and the pressure rose, he slipped into a coma and died.

Then, in the 1960s, Dr. Long began working with a fellow Minnesota neurosurgeon, Dr. Joseph Galicich, who first demonstrated that high doses of the new steroid drugs could dramatically reduce brain swelling. Suddenly, surgeons were able to try far more extensive surgery, and to operate on previously inoperable patients. Dr. Long's work in steroid therapy was one of the principal reasons he was chosen to occupy the Harvey Cushing Chair.

But when the television networks invite Dr. Long to appear on their morning talk shows, when important groups around the world ask him to come and give a speech, when newspaper correspondents interview him . . . do they want to talk about steroid therapy? What is steroid therapy? Who cares?

But pain, like the soul, is universal. It's something everybody understands.

Over the years, Dr. Long managed to reduce his pain practice. But he was still obligated, as the expert, to supervise and participate. He was obligated, by his calculations, every third month. This day, he would far rather have been in the operating room helping Dr. Murray remove Joe Trott's acoustic tumor. Instead, he gathered up his papers and headed toward the old conference room on Brady One.

On his way he stopped at a doctors' lunchroom and picked up a tuna salad sandwich to take with him. Carrying his sandwich, his mind on Joe Trott, Dr. Long rode down an elevator to the second floor, zigzagged through a series of hallways, and cut through the Halsted building and the Children's Medical and Surgical Center. Then, having reached Brady Two, he walked down polished white marble steps to the Chronic Pain Treatment Center.

He was met in the center by Dr. Nelson Hendler, the consulting psychiatrist, and four nurses, a physical therapist, a psychiatric aide and a neurosurgical resident. They all had their lunches with them. While they ate, they chatted about general pain clinic matters.

When he finished his sandwich, Dr. Long leaned back and reached out toward the rack of patient charts behind him. He opened the first one.

"Mrs. Walker is fifty-four," he said, "and a longtime patient at Johns Hopkins. Her complaint is of neck and jaw pain. She says she was lifting something—a sack of kitty litter, I believe—when something snapped in her neck. The X-rays were negative. She was put in traction, and she says the traction dislocated her neck."

One of the nurses glanced up from her notes. "She doesn't show any nonverbal pain behavior, but she talks about it constantly. She doesn't think we believe her."

Dr. Long smiled. "Perceptive lady."

Her complaint, the chief neurosurgeon said, is anatomically impossible. The brain simply isn't wired in such a way as to combine the variety of complaints the patient has. She can't, for instance, have pain in one side of her face, and the same side of her body. The patient probably doesn't know that the brain is crosswired below the neck. If her problem was caused by a lesion in the nervous system, then it would be in one side of her face and the *opposite* side of her body.

"I have a notion," he said, "that we will find deep-seated psychological problems."

Dr. Hendler, the psychiatrist, nodded assent. "I saw evidence of some deep familial scars." He added that he intended to schedule her for a truth serum interview, which sometimes helped identify the problem. Once the doctors knew what the lizard brain was trying to do, they could often figure out how to stop it.

The ring of a wall phone near the door interrupted the conversation. Dr. Long's attention went instantly to the telephone, and the nurse who had answered it.

The nurse listened for a moment, and then shook her head negatively at Dr. Long. No, it wasn't Dr. Murray calling from the OR.

Dr. Long brought his mind back to the pain problem and reached for the next chart.

"Mary Sanders," he read aloud, "thirty-eight, divorced, three children, total body pain, no physical findings . . ."

CHAPTER
ELEVEN

In Operating Room Eleven, Dr. Murray squinted through the eyepieces of the operating microscope, examining the tumor up close. The scrub nurse was busy laying out a kit of tiny, long-handled tools. Each went in its traditional place, a place the nurse's fingers knew by rote.

The instruments were made primarily of titanium, to minimize their weight. Their tips were as tiny, and as fragile, as watchmakers' tools. There were diminutive hooks, scissors, knives, bludgeons and probes, and they were very expensive. The prices started at perhaps one hundred dollars, and the nurse handled them with care.

In a few minutes, without looking up from the microscope, Dr. Murray called for a micro-scalpel. For a moment, he held it in his hand by the very tip, balancing it. He changed its position slightly. Now, it felt comfortable.

The surgeon's eyes stayed pressed against the eyepieces. His assistant guided his hand and the scalpel safely to the hole in Joe's head, keeping it well clear of the aye-ka. He released Dr. Murray's hand when the tip of the instrument swam into the microscopic field.

For a moment, the scalpel rested high against the wall of the tumor. Then, glinting in the microscope's headlight, it moved downward. The tumor membrane separated cleanly, revealing a yellow, gristly-looking mass about the consistency of cottage cheese. Unlike brain tissue, it didn't tend to pour out through the slit in its membrane.

The scalpel disappeared, and in a moment the jaws of a nipper swam into view. The nipper jockeyed for position, then clamped down over a bit of tumor tissue and bit it free.

Dr. Murray removed the biopsy cutter from the hole and dropped the sample into the nurse's gloved hand. She placed it in a vial and handed it to a waiting attendant from the pathology lab. He took it and disappeared.

It would greatly surprise Dr. Murray to discover that Joe's tumor was malignant. But if it was, he'd rather be surprised now than later.

Assuming it wasn't cancerous, he and Dr. Long would go for a cure, for total removal of the tumor. There was a small but very real possibility that, in the process, they would kill Joe.

By the look of it, the tumor was wrapped around the basilar artery and, since it was an acoustic tumor, it was probably stuck tightly.

The basilar artery was one of the three big feeder arteries of the brain. If it were torn, it would squirt blood all the way out to the objective lens of the microscope. Joe would die.

If the tumor wasn't cancerous, the risk was balanced with the prospect of a long, normal life for the patient. Joe was young, with a bright future. If they got all the tumor, it wouldn't grow back. It would be worth going for broke.

But if the thing was cancerous, it would recur no matter how heroic the surgeons' efforts. If death would come anyway in a few months, scraping the tumor off the basilar wouldn't make any difference. So why risk what little life Joe would have left?

But Dr. Murray was certain it wouldn't come to that. After fifteen years in neurosurgery, he figured he knew a noncancerous tumor when he saw one.

Not bothering to wait for the pathology report, he called for the microsucker, and used it to probe at the guts of the thing. Under the slight pressure of the sucker, the yellow flesh moved back and forth, ever so gently.

Dr. Murray kept the suction low, so that the sucker didn't really tug, more of an urging, urging, moving back and forth across its surface, brushing it, the suction sort of wearing away at it with nudges and hints.

Remembering the haze of blood vessels on the angiogram, Dr. Murray stopped and studied the eroding face of the tumor. If they are seen in time, the bleeders can be burned closed and then cut away. If not seen in time, the sucker would wear away a vessel wall and suddenly there would be blood all over the field and quiet terror in the OR.

Under the high magnification, the spurting vessel would seem huge, and its severed end would sometimes whip around like a runaway fire hose. It was unthinkable, but nonetheless possible, that in the excitement, while looking for the severed end, or trying to grab it with the bipolars, a luckless surgeon might forget exactly where he was in relation to the aye-ka.

Dr. Murray moved slowly, carefully, sucking, teasing, urging, watching for bleeders, finding them, and burning them shut. Slowly, the sucker pulled away layer after layer of cells until an indentation appeared in the yellow wall. As the minutes passed, the indentation deepened and became a tunnel.

The pathologist stuck his head through the doorway. *Schwannoma,* he said. *Acoustic tumor.*

Dr. Murray looked up. He had thought so, but, still . . . smile wrinkles appeared above his mask. Then he went back to work.

Patiently, the neurosurgeon eroded his way into the tumor. The minute hand of the clock moved steadily. The monitors beeped. The anesthesiologist leaned back in his chair, his eyes focused on his rhythmically moving dials.

One resident stood at the side 'scope, assisting, and a more junior man stood well back, his eyes on the television monitor. As he worked, Dr. Murray talked to them.

There is a trick in debulking a tumor like this, he explained. You make a tunnel into it and then, with a little bit of teasing, let the roof of the tunnel fall down onto you. Clear that aside and nudge, touch, urge a wall to collapse. Suck away the rubble. Undermine the other wall. Slowly, as you work, the tumor will collapse down around you, and that way, you were always working in the middle of the tumor, at a maximum distance from the gray neurons.

You also had to keep in mind as you worked that Joe's tumor was a big one, and, as it grew, it had pushed normal structures aside. Even the brain stem can be bent, if it's done slowly, over months or years.

Now, in the course of a very few hours, the pressure would be relieved and the stem would settle back, an eighth of an inch, a quarter of an inch—a huge distance for such a delicate structure to move so rapidly. Such a motion could kill cells.

Your first warning might be that the heart would slow, or begin to race. The lesson was that when you so much as touched one part of the brain you affected all of it. His sucker, now, was a full inch from the brain stem, but you had to remember . . .

In the anesthesiologist's cockpit the dials jumped and the lights flashed. The steady beep, beep, beeping of the heart monitor was backed up by a softer, almost inaudible ka-GLUP, ka-GLUP, ka-GLUP, the direct sound of the heart pumping. Perfect.

Slowly. Time and patience.

Not pulling, tugging, except not quite tugging, urging. By watching the television screen, the scrub nurse followed the operation, anticipating which tools Dr. Murray would call for.

Suction.
Cotton ball.
Microscissors.
Suction.
Irrigation.
Suction.
Bayonet.
The aye-ka is right there.
Cotton ball.
Beep, beep, beep, beep, beep, beep.
As he worked, Dr. Murray discovered that the tumor had grown around and enveloped many of the structures at the bottom of the skull cavity. Several important cranial nerves had been engulfed by the growing tumor.

Now those vital communication links were tubes of softness running through the mushy tumor. If the suction tube blundered into one of them, part of Joe's head and face would be paralyzed. Dr. Murray stared into the eyepieces, carefully scrutinizing the field.

Under the microscope, the thing was a mountain, far too big to see all at once.

The buzzing, Joe said, had been in the left ear, so the tumor probably sprouted originally from the left auditory nerve. That nerve, by now, must be completely destroyed. The neurosurgeons could save Joe's life, but they couldn't give him back hearing in his left ear.

It was a wonder how long some patients could put off coming to a doctor. Joe was lucky. A few years ago, a patient in his condition would have been as good as dead.

Carefully, Dr. Murray moved the microsuction device back and forth, back and forth, across the face of the tunnel.

The surgeon and his assistant bent, almost immobile, above the microscope. The scrub nurse stood poised, unblinking. The circulating nurse leaned against a stainless-steel cabinet, beneath the face of the clock.

The best way to operate on the brain was not to touch it.

In the adjacent operating room, a mop bucket clattered. That case was finished, apparently. But Dr. Murray was just getting started.

Three buildings and seven floors away, pain rounds drew to a close. The therapists gathered up their notes. Dr. Long replaced the last chart in the rack, stood up, went to the wall phone, and dialed Fran's number.

"No sir, Dr. Murray hasn't called."

Very good. That meant everything was still fine.

Dr. Long thought a minute. He really should go to grand rounds. He would rather be in the OR, but the chief neurosurgeon should definitely go to grand rounds. Yes. He'd better go, and stay as long as possible.

Yes sir, Fran said. She noted the new number and promised to call him the instant she heard from Dr. Murray in the OR.

Alerts and Red Alerts were part of Dr. Long's life. Though he had collected a cadre of highly skilled neurosurgeons to run his department, he remained the most experienced, and he was the one they called when they had something interesting or when Something Awful happened in the operating room.

The last time he was called for Something Awful was several months ago. He was preparing to leave for home, wife, children, garden, maybe a cup of Red Rose tea in front of the fireplace. The intercom called his name as he strolled through the hallway toward the parking garage.

Big Red was in OR 11. Dr. Long didn't even have time to scrub.

The nurses draped a sterile gown over his street clothes and he pulled a pair of sterile gloves over his hands. The frightened younger surgeon who had been operating stepped willingly, gratefully, to the side microscope.

Methodically, refusing to panic, Dr. Long fished through the sea of churning blood.

"Irrigation."

"Suction."

The water swirled into the surgical hole, and the opaque red blood turned pink. It disappeared into the suction hose and then, for a moment, Dr. Long could see the direction of the flow. Then the hole was filled again with blood. The first problem was to find out where the blood was coming from.

"Irrigation. Suction." His voice was calm, almost flat—his high-tension voice.

The flow was coming from the right quadrant of the hole, he decided. The next time he had a moment to glimpse, he narrowed the possibilities. In the course of his career, Dr. Long had also picked up a degree in neuroanatomy. At times like these, it helped.

Finally he located the source of the blood, clamped it off. The younger surgeon, shaken and grateful, helped him repair the damage. The patient lived.

If Dr. Murray ran into trouble, Fran always knew where Dr. Long could be reached.

Now, pain rounds finished, Dr. Long walked quickly toward the auditorium in the faraway Wilmer building.

He would have rather been in OR 11 with Dr. Murray, but it was especially important, these days, for him to attend grand rounds. He had a Great Experiment going with grand rounds.

Grand rounds were quite different from ordinary, bedside rounds. Bedside rounds occurred twice a day, every day of the year, including Christmas. A senior doctor, accompanied by an entourage of junior ones, went from bed to bed. The senior man discussed each case and bombarded the residents with questions. Bedside rounds were informal and very practical, and followed a tradition that has been handed down to successive generations of doctors since the Middle Ages.

Grand rounds, in contrast, were a formal and, from a resident's viewpoint, formidable occasion.

Grand rounds convened in a teaching hall, where the patients were discussed in absentia. Each resident went to the front of the room to discuss his cases. The senior men sat in the audience, criticized, and asked knowing and sometimes loaded questions.

Traditionally, each of the various specialties on the brain met separately for grand rounds. The neurosurgeons, the neurologists and the psychiatrists were all concerned with the same organ, the brain, but, oddly, they had little to say to one another.

Psychiatrists, an old saying goes, don't know anything about the brain and couldn't do anything about it if they did. Neurologists know everything about the brain but can't do anything about it. Neurosurgeons know nothing about the brain—but will try anything.

The saying sums up an old attitude that had its roots in experience as well as prejudice.

The forces that dominated the psychiatrist's world were vastly different from those of the neurologist, and the neurologist's problems were fundamentally different from the neurosurgeon's. The specialties used radically different methods to treat different diseases in different patients. This gave each profession its own perspective, and each doctor naturally saw his own role as the most interesting.

From the neurosurgical point of view, the neurologist was a sort of detective. The neurologist examined the patient and noted the symptoms. Perhaps there was a numbness of the left side of the face, increasing deafness in the left ear, a marked lack of co-ordination and, finally, double vision beginning in the lower left field. The neurologist ruminated on that for a while, rummaged around in books, maybe, and deduced a tumor in the posterior fossa. In effect, his business was to tell the neurosurgeon where to make the incision.

The neurologist, understandably, tended to allot himself a more central role in the hospital drama. They called him for stroke patients, and overdose cases, and aneurysms, and weird, puzzling conditions like premature senility.

And, they reminded one another, their voices reflecting the horror they felt, remember neurosurgery's favorite way of removing a tumor? You stuck your thumb in the thing, and popped it right out! Just the thought was enough to make a neurologist shudder.

It was only natural that, over the generations, neurologists developed a certain disdain for the neurosurgeon and his clumsy, bloody craft. A neurologist felt somehow guilty when he turned a patient over to a neurosurgeon.

But the realities dividing neurosurgery and neurology had been modified in recent years. With the advent of the CAT-scanner the neurologist no longer had so much detective work to do for the surgeons. An amateur could find a tumor on a CAT scan.

At the same time, neurologists were discovering how to manipulate the brain chemically, as well as diagnose it. As the 1980s opened, they were busy treating patients who, not many years before, would have been hopeless. It was no longer true that neurologists could do nothing, and their defensiveness waned.

The neurosurgeons, in the meantime, aided by the microscope, came to understand the brain on an ever finer scale. The thumb-pop method of tumor removal fell into disfavor, and then disuse. Neurosurgeons tried to forget it had ever been done that way.

Then came the steroid drugs to prevent swelling, and that changed everything. The neurologists, when referring patients to neurosurgery, no longer had to think of themselves as pronouncing a death sentence.

The time had come, Dr. Long thought, for neurologists and neurosurgeons to start communicating more directly. The chief of neurology agreed, and they hesitantly, rather tentatively, took the revolutionary step of combining neurological and neurosurgical grand rounds. That was why Dr. Long really needed to attend, if he could. A chief of neurosurgery has political duties, too.

Today, Dr. Long stood toward the back, contributing occasionally but remaining near the telephone. One after the other, the residents slowly mounted the stage and chanted their patient notes into the microphone.

Dr. Long kept looking at his watch. An hour passed, and the telephone didn't ring. Once he reached out, as though to pick it up, and then changed his mind. Fran would call.

Finally, an instant before the last resident finished his presentation, before somebody could buttonhole him, Dr. Long slipped out the door. His hands in the pockets of his white smock, he walked quickly down the long hallway between the buildings.

Outside, it was a gray day. The ground was thawed by now, but still too cold for seed.

Dr. Long changed into his scrub suit in the professors' locker room, and snatched a paper cap and a mask out of the dispenser. He went down the flight of stairs quickly.

It was 3 P.M. when Dr. Long entered the operating room. Dr. Murray lifted his eyes from the microscope and straightened up, flexing his back and shoulders.

"You're just in time," he said.

Dr. Murray explained that he had excavated three quarters of the tumor's mass from the inside. The tumor had collapsed inward, as expected. As the pressure on the brain stem lessened, it had presumably sagged back toward its normal position, but there had been no problems. The heartbeat, as Dr. Long could tell by listening, was strong and steady.

Dr. Long moved up to the main 'scope and Dr. Murray took the position to the side. As his chief scanned the landscape, he pointed out the damp cotton pad to one side of the wound. The aye-ka was right there, under the cotton.

The yellow tissue dominated the center of the deep hole in Joe Trott's head. Looking up over the partially collapsed tumor, Dr. Long could see the upper part of the brain stem, a structure called the pons.

But the lower brain stem disappeared behind the tumor and, life being what it was, the tumor capsule would probably be stuck to it.

With luck, it would not be stuck too tightly.

The key, he told Dr. Murray and the two residents, would be finding a cleavage plane. A cleavage plane was an area of natural separation between two materials. The segments of an orange, for instance, were separated by cleavage planes.

If he could find a plane, the tumor membrane should peel back across the top of the tumor and down alongside the brain stem.

The gelatinous tissue of the brain stem bulged downward behind its thin membranes, throbbing and heaving with each heartbeat.

Even with a cleavage plane, you couldn't just pull the tumor loose, of course. You didn't even think about doing that. You could push at it, not push, poke, not poke, nudge, suggest . . . beckon . . .

As Dr. Long worked at the tumor, Dr. Murray flexed his muscles.

Neurosurgeons can train themselves to ignore a full bladder, but the muscles in the small of the back and the shoulders won't be ignored. While he was operating, Dr. Murray didn't notice the pain. But as soon as he stepped back, ouch, ouch, ouch. At a hospital like Hopkins, ten- and twelve-hour operations were common, but not common enough that you ever got used to them. Dr. Murray longed for a quiet, suburban practice.

Dr. Long, his muscles fresh and his mind clear, was immediately absorbed by the problem before him. Gently, he worried at the tumor membrane. The ceiling jiggled and pulsed.

Sometimes, removing a tightly stuck tumor capsule could be like trying to peel an unco-operative boiled egg. The inside of the egg stuck to the shell, and when you peeled it, unless you were very careful, hunks of egg white came off with the shell.

Joe Trott's brain was softer than boiled egg white, though. And you could throw away an egg.

Dr. Long poked at the tumor, worried with it, and then stepped back a moment to think.

Rotten luck. It was stuck to everything!

A moment later he moved back to the microscope, the sucker in his hand. Patiently, he teased, urged, suggested, beckoned the tattered yellow tissue. It obeyed, but slowly and stubbornly, as the suction tool moved back and forth.

Control of the sucker was an art in itself. It had an extra hole where it fit into the surgeon's hand. If the surgeon didn't put a finger over that hole, the suction would all be lost. If the hole was covered, the sucker would pull with full force. A skilled surgeon could, by moving his finger slightly, exercise precise control over the amount of suction being used.

To be gentle, Dr. Long shifted his finger slightly, and let some of the suction be lost. Gently, gently, gently, he teased at the membrane with the sucker tip, gently, gently, pulling away the diseased flesh.

Slowly, slowly . . . too slowly. Dr. Long glanced at the clock.

Joe had been on the table nine hours. That was a worry. It would be best to get this over with quickly, but, so far, Dr. Long had not found a plane.

He could hurry things, but he didn't dare. If he tried to hurry, the beckon might become a tug, and the delicate membranes might shear, and then Joe would vanish.

If only he could find a separation plane. But none appeared.

The monitor continued steady, beep, beep, beep . . .

The scrub nurse's eyes were fixed on the television monitor.

The blunt, flattened end of a microdissector replaced the sucker and moved ponderously across the field, huge under fifteen magnifications. The lizard brain glittered wetly.

Finally Dr. Long stepped back. This was not working.

He would try another approach, maybe find a plane. He would go down to the right, where the aye-ka snaked back behind the tumor, leading to the basilar artery.

Thoughtfully, he repositioned the microscope, then reached out his hand for the sucker.

Gently . . . probing, sucking, worrying, suggesting. The minutes passed.

A nurse counted bloody gauze sponges and tied them neatly in bundles of ten. Out in the hallway, an OR crew wheeled an emergency case toward another operating room. An autoclave hissed.

Working along the bottom of the tumor, Dr. Long found the ninth, tenth and eleventh cranial nerves and noted where they disappeared into the tumor capsule. Carefully, the surgeon nudged the tumor surface, and it moved. The nerve moved, too. It was stuck tight.

He teased, urged, beckoned.

Nothing.

Careful, or Joe will never taste another watermelon. Easy, or he'll be unable to move his head to look at a pretty girl. Gently, or Joe will be unable to swallow, and will eventually choke to death.

Delicately, delicately, Dr. Long teased. Finally, the tumor began to peel back. The scrub nurse waited, immobile. The hands of the clock turned, too slowly to watch.

The anesthesiologist reached for his clipboard.

Then he froze.

Beep, beep, beep . . . beep . . . beep . . . beep.

Bradycardia. Something was happening. The heart was slowing down.

With the heart's first hesitation, Dr. Long's instruments instantly ceased to move. Then, carefully, they withdrew.

The senior surgeon looked at the clock. 5:59.

Beep . . . beep . . . beep . . .

Decision. Leave the tumor capsule where it is, for now. Come back another day.

This tumor is stuck to everything. Don't try it today. Return when the patient is fresh, and stronger. Retreat while Joe is alive.

The microscope swung back, and the overhead lights came on. Blinking in the sudden brightness, Dr. Murray moved in to oversee the closure.

Joe, Dr. Long knew, would be plenty angry. But there was no other rational choice.

As he left the operating room, the chief of neurosurgery stripped the rubber gloves from his hands and dropped them in a trash can.

CHAPTER
TWELVE

RICHARD THOUGHT ABOUT THE SCHIZOPHRENIC AS HE WALKED OUT TO THE parking lot, unlocked his Camaro and drove home. The man had been abjectly grateful for his shower. He had said thank you, thank you, thank you, over and over again. Richard wondered. Was there a chemical for gratitude?

Whatever it was, Richard knew the feeling, knew the awful self-hatred of having failed again, having become crazy again. He knew the feeling too well, and took his responsibilities at the clinic too seriously, to be able to forget about work when he walked out the clinic's front door. Besides, you can't be a forty-hour-a-week man and get anywhere in life, and have your kid go to college.

Since it was almost midnight and the traffic was light, it took him only fifteen minutes to get to the apartment. As he pulled into the parking place by the dumpster, a rat's eyes glittered briefly in his headlights, but Richard didn't notice.

He kept his mind firmly fixed on his new patient, ignoring the dirty streets, the three young men on the corner under the streetlights, the Communist slogan painted on the wall of his hallway. Those things represented the outside world, the one he had resolved to rise above. He had decided long ago that they were best ignored.

The frontier between inside and outside was his front door. It had three locks.

He opened the door, kissed his pregnant wife, and waved a greeting at his brother, who was sitting on the couch. The door closed, the locks snapped, and Richard kicked off his shoes. He walked through the spotless living room and into the kitchen.

The 7-Up didn't hiss when he opened it, and it was almost gone. Damn. He would have to go out.

In the car, Richard bantered briefly with his brother about the University of Maryland basketball team, and then he fell silent. His mind wandered back, automatically, and he was sitting in the day room with the schizophrenic, after the shower.

He'd talked to the man about how you had to take care of your mind, have mental hygiene—you know, the same way you keep your toenails clean.

He had thought the patient was paying attention, but then he'd noticed the blinking. The man was blinking, but it wasn't like a real blinking, it was . . . different. The eyelids would snap down, just once. Then the head would turn, and they would snap down again.

"What are you doing?" Richard asked.

"I'm taking pictures," the man replied. "I want a record of this."

Classic schizophrenia.

Too much dopamine in the lizard brain. Or was it too little dopamine? Suddenly, Richard couldn't remember. Or was it serotonin?

The fast-foods place was right ahead. He could see the big plastic sign on the high pole. It was close, but it seemed somehow . . . distant.

Dopamine? Or serotonin?

Irritated, Richard tried to focus his mind. He'd studied that just . . . yesterday?

Or was it the day before that?

His brother asked him something, mumbled. It didn't seem important. Richard concentrated on his driving. It took a lot more energy to drive than he remembered.

His fingertips and toes felt numb, and his chest didn't want to suck in air. He could barely feel the wheel enough to turn the car into the parking lot. His right foot wouldn't work. He touched the power-brake with his left and the Camaro jerked to a halt in front of the convenience store.

Serotonin? Or dopamine? Which?

Why wouldn't his head work?

He pulled himself out of the car, and it took a great effort. He was so tired, and his body didn't want to stand. He leaned on the car and saw his brother looking back at him across the roof.

His brother looked funny, surprised, sort of. Helpless. Like something didn't make sense.

Richard turned and forced himself to walk, pitted himself against the unresponsive muscles, and lurched forward, dragging his right side.

Time was syrupy. People were looking at him.

He opened the glass door and made his way toward the soft-drink cooler. The damned refrigerator door wouldn't open, no, the arm wouldn't reach for it. He looked down. The fingers curled back, then forward, making a claw. A claw with clean fingernails. A dead claw, not part of Richard at all.

7-Up. He was here for 7-Up.

Green bottle. Cold.

Glass case.

The fingers of Richard's left hand wrapped around the neck of the 7-Up bottle.

Pay. Pay the woman.

He hopped to the counter on his left foot. The cashier waited on him quickly, then stepped back. She seemed afraid.

Richard's brother put his arm around his chest and helped him outside and into the passenger side of the car. His brother wanted the keys, but Richard couldn't make himself respond, couldn't make himself care. He felt his brother's hand in his pocket.

The car moved slowly, at first, then faster, like his brother was in a hurry. Richard saw it all from far, far away.

At home, when he couldn't get out of the car, his brother lifted him out and carried him up the steps of his apartment. Inside, his wife rushed to the telephone.

Richard lay on the couch and stared at the ceiling. After a while there were a lot of people in the room, and several hands transferred him to a stretcher.

Richard's mind recorded the red and white flashing lights. It took him back, back, where he didn't want to go, to the hateful ghetto.

Sometimes there'd be an overdose, or a knifing, or someone would hang himself with a belt or a piece of sheet. Sometimes there were blue lights, too. Blue lights meant police. There weren't any blue lights now, though.

The schizophrenic's blinking, picture-taking eyes floated into Richard's mind.

He remembered walking down the hall, the man plucking at his sleeve. Richard knew what it was like to have somebody help, to get another chance, and to be grateful. Thank you, the man had said, wretched in his helplessness.

In the ambulance, the medic saw Richard's lips move, and he bent over to hear.

"Thank you," Richard murmured. "Thank you, thank you, thank you . . ."

"You're gonna be all right, man," the medic said, automatically grabbing a handhold as the vehicle lurched, siren howling, onto the dark street.

CHAPTER
THIRTEEN

SOMEWHERE, IT WAS WARM.

Down in St. Thomas the sun was shining and sailboats cut across the warm blue surface of the Carribean. Music floated up from below decks, and there was the laughter of women and children. If Tom Ducker were there, he would stretch out behind the wheel, in the shadow of the mains'l, and . . .

But Tom Ducker wasn't there.

Tom Ducker was sitting behind a desk on the twelfth floor of University Hospital. It was midmorning. The patients had been seen, the letters had been signed, the telephone calls had been returned and the desk was clean. He pushed back his chair, then hesitated.

It would be cold, in the big walk-in deep-freeze.

The thought came and disappeared, and the neurosurgeon rose to his feet. It didn't help to put things off. Quite the contrary, procrastination often made things worse.

On the way out he told Barbara Burns, his secretary, that he would be in the lab doing squirrels for the next couple of hours. Outside in the hallway he paced in front of the elevator door.

The problem with doing surgery in a refrigerator was that very few surgeons besides Tom Ducker did it. Thus there was no market for, say, insulated surgical gloves. The first few times he operated in the deep freeze, Tom Ducker damn near froze his fingers off. His toes, too.

It had all begun in Italy at one of those big international scientific meetings. Tom Ducker had been perusing the conference schedule, and he discovered, to his surprise, that one of the speakers was a scientist from another part of the big University of Maryland Medical School campus. Dr. Ducker didn't know the fellow, except slightly, by reputation. It seemed silly to travel halfway across the world to hear a Maryland scientist speak, but, still . . . a hunch flitted across the neurosurgeon's mind. Why not? On a whim, Dr. Ducker went to hear Dr. Edson Albuquerque present his paper.

Dr. Albuquerque was a specialist in the physiology of brain cells, and the symposium in which he spoke dealt with theoretical ways of tricking the gray neurons into reproducing.

Dr. Ducker knew the problem better than most, since he spent a large part of his time treating accident victims in the University of Maryland's shock-trauma unit. Damaged brains and spinal cords didn't recover, no matter how carefully he treated them, and he knew first-hand the tragedy of brain-damaged fathers and quadriplegic teenagers.

He listened to the panel of scientists speak, one after another. When it was Dr. Albuquerque's turn, he mounted the stand and told the audience that he and a colleague, Dr. Lloyd Guth, had found evidence that hibernating squirrels might be able to regenerate damaged spinal cords.

The audience, in Dr. Ducker's opinion, seemed to discount the possibility. It did sound like a rather incredible claim. Either the fellow was a dunce . . . or he was on to something big.

The hunch that had brought the neurosurgeon to the session grew more powerful as the morning proceeded. When the meeting broke up, he approached Dr. Albuquerque and offered his services.

A few months later, he started spending an occasional morning in the deep freeze, severing the spinal cords of hibernating squirrels. The squirrels were kept in the freezer for a time, after surgery, and then put in a warm room. Their back legs were paralyzed, of course.

Then they were watched, carefully, to see if they regained any use of those legs.

Tom Ducker's part of it was minor, but nonetheless necessary. The spinal cords had to be completely severed by a surgeon who would put his reputation on the line in attesting to that fact. Otherwise, if one of the squirrels regained some use of his back legs, there would be lingering doubt. Scientists, always skeptical, would wonder whether the spinal cord had only been incompletely severed.

Like most bright new ideas in science, the hibernating squirrel project would probably yield nothing. But if it did, it would be the most important discovery in neurosurgery since Harvey Cushing discovered that you could enter the posterior fossa without killing the patient. If one of the squirrels regained its ability to walk, someone would go to Sweden to pick up a Nobel.

It wouldn't be Tom Ducker, though. His part was too minor. The closest this project was going to get him to Stockholm was the Swedish boot-liners he'd scrounged up to wear in the deep freeze.

Actually, they helped a lot. They were made of thick felt, and they reached all the way to his knees, and he hadn't had cold feet in the freezer. He just wished he could think of something as effective to protect his hands. The thin latex surgical gloves offered no protection at all to his fingers.

In a laboratory area a few feet from the freezer door, Dr. Ducker undressed, put on long underpants and a sweater, and donned a scrub suit. His feet slipped easily into the big mukluks.

He wished it were spring.

He pulled hard against the big freezer door, and it swung slowly open. A technician came behind him, and closed it again.

The far end of the freezer was occupied by shelves of plastic cages, each of them occupied by a hibernating squirrel. A tiny surgical table was set up by the door. Dr. Ducker sat down on a stool in front of it, and got right to work adjusting the small operating microscope. The sooner he got started, the sooner he would be done.

There would be three squirrels, today. Earlier the assistant had moved their cages over next to the operating table, and now he placed the first one in front of the neurosurgeon. The squirrel was brown, with a double black stripe down its back. It lay curled tightly in the fetal position, its nose nestled against its belly and its tail curling up over its head.

With each exhaled breath, fog drifted from beneath the men's surgical masks. Dr. Ducker straightened the squirrel out and held it tightly as the assistant clipped the hair from a little patch of the animal's back, just behind the shoulder blades. Already, Dr. Ducker could feel the chill spreading through his fingers, reducing their dexterity.

It was probably colder in the freezer than it was outside.

In theory, of course, you could sail the Chesapeake in this weather. It was a protected body of water, and this late in the winter there usually wasn't much ice. Several times, in desperation, Dr. Ducker had tried it. But there were limits. Tom Ducker wasn't a fanatic, and didn't want to be one. So he contented himself with playing squash in the winter.

But God, he wished it were spring.

He took a hypodermic syringe from the assistant and quickly injected a local anesthetic around the clipped spot on the squirrel's back. The animal wriggled groggily, then went back to sleep.

One thing a neurosurgeon learned, early in his career, was that you needed something, something different, something free, like tacking into a September breeze, the Chesapeake Bay Bridge on the horizon, an eye to a distant bank of clouds, wind howling through the slot, deck tilted at a forty-five-degree angle, wheel firmly in his hands . . . you needed that, or something like it.

If you didn't have it, you might find you didn't have what it took to go into the operating room. If you didn't have it, you might try to find it in a bottle, or in ego, and then you might touch something that shouldn't be disturbed, and someone might die.

Donlin Long, over at the Hopkins, had his garden, and it brought him peace. Michael Salcman . . .

Michael Salcman was a New York boy, and New York was at least as far from Tom Ducker's West Virginia as, say, New Delhi. The two could talk about such things as baseball and neurosurgical approaches, but in other ways their interests and experiences diverged.

Michael had firm opinions about the opera, for instance. He wrote poetry, and he and his wife Ilene spent considerable time poking through modern art galleries. He talked about such things with great enthusiasm, and on such occasions Tom Ducker remained silent.

He didn't really understand the modern paintings that Michael collected. He could understand a painting of a person, or a meadow, or a sailboat, but he didn't have a feel for nonrepresentational shapes, and things that looked like splatters on canvas. At the same time, he could tell that Michael did, and he could recognize the function of an art collection.

It was a different kind of joy, apparently, but Tom Ducker could tell that his junior colleague took something important from his art collection, something indefinable, something in some mute way not unlike what he, Tom Ducker, took from sailing.

And Michael's art collection had one huge advantage over Tom Ducker's sailboat and Donlin Long's garden. In the winter Tom Ducker had to content himself with squash, and Donlin Long was forced to fall back on seed catalogs. But Michael could collect art, and enjoy it, all year round.

Dr. Ducker reached out for a scalpel, and the laboratory technician put it in his hand. The blade glinted in the bright light as the neurosurgeon carefully parted the skin over the squirrel's spine. There was almost no blood; a hibernating squirrel's heart beats only about once a minute.

Working quickly but carefully, Dr. Ducker used a tiny nipper to bite away the top of a vertebra. Below lay the spinal cord. The operating microscope swung into place.

After introducing himself to Dr. Albuquerque at that faraway meeting, Dr. Ducker returned home and thought the theory over.

The central nervous system didn't repair itself, scientists had always assumed, because, well, because it didn't. Perhaps the genetic code in the neuron's chromosomes had been converted to memory molecules, and the brain cell couldn't reproduce. Perhaps . . . anything. Whatever the reason, it was somehow fitting that such a delicate organ would be unrepairable, but until recently, few scientists thought about it much.

But now . . . given time, perhaps the nerve cells *could* regenerate, or at least grow new connections. Perhaps the servant cells, in their haste to build a scar around the wound, prevented the tiny axons from making new connections. That was analogous to what happened in the peripheral nervous system, in an injured nerve—as with Josh's crippled hand.

Dr. Albuquerque had observed that the glial cells were especially crippled by cold, and that brain and spinal cord scars didn't form so readily in hibernating animals. That might, then, give the neurons a chance to send out new axons, and to make new connections.

Dr. Ducker focused the microscope onto the squirrel's exposed spinal cord. With the tip of the scalpel, he sliced through the cord, using a back-and-forth motion to be sure it was completely cut. Afterward he examined the cut ends carefully, to make certain he had severed every last nerve pathway.

Then, patiently, as patiently as he had repaired the ulnar nerve in Josh's arm, he used a tiny needle and sutures too small to see with the naked eye, and sewed the spinal cord back together.

It was cold, cold in the freezer. It was cold outside. Too cold, far too cold, to sail.

To be a first-rate sailor, you had to be in sympathy with nature, had to know intimately the forces you harnessed, and how they behaved. If you were good enough, and skillful enough, you could turn the breeze and the sea to your own uses, and you could foil nature, and trick it into blowing you upwind.

But in sailing, as in neurosurgery, something could always happen. And when it did, it tested you. Like the time off Long Island.

Tom had been in college then, and was spending the summer as a sailing instructor and harbor master at a yacht club on Long Island Sound.

He was a highly competent sailor, even then, though he hadn't been tested. As he taught others to sail, his own skills improved, and by that summer he handled a boat with easy confidence—no wasted motions, no false moves.

When a group of businessmen wanted to sail their forty-two-foot yacht in a regatta, he was the obvious one to approach. Would he captain the boat, with them as crew?

A beautiful boat like that? Tom didn't hesitate. Of course he would. Besides, he had never won a regatta. Maybe this time . . .

The storm had appeared without warning, unheralded by the weather forecasters. The clouds gathered, the winds picked up to gale force, the sea heaved and frothed and came slamming into the hull. In minutes, a pleasant sail turned ominous, then frightening. Suddenly the coastline seemed far away.

Tom fought the wheel, keeping the boat from being broadsided and capsized by the waves, and shouted orders into the wind. The businessmen tried desperately to reef in the mains'l, but they lacked the skill. The gale pulled the lines from their fingers and the sail was snatched aloft, booming and cracking against the rigging, tearing itself apart. The terrified businessmen fled below decks.

Alone in the cockpit, Tom kept one hand on the wheel and used the other to lash a length of rope around his waist and tie himself to the mizzenmast behind him. With only a storm jib aloft and functioning, he fought to avoid being swamped.

He fought the storm for hours, desperately struggling to keep the boat from drifting broadside to the crashing waves. The wind tore the tops from the waves, sending water flying horizontally, like a salty rain that pelted against his face. Wave after wave slammed into the stern, lifting the boat high and then letting it crash down, wallowing, in the trough that followed. There, in the momentary calm, he could hear the businessmen being seasick below.

Occasionally, during the long hours, the businessmen pleaded with Tom to save their lives. The boat didn't matter, they said. If he got them back to shore, he could have the damned boat.

Finally the gale died and the waves fell, and Tom sailed the boat back into the marina. By that time, the businessmen had recovered enough to swagger around the decks and boast of the storm they had conquered. They forgot their offer to give Tom the boat.

But they were right. The boat didn't matter. The storm had tested Tom, and had not found him wanting. What's more, he had not only finished the regatta, he had placed second.

Soon after, Tom Ducker won his first regatta.

Much later, when he became a neurosurgeon, he quit sailing competitively. After a week in the operating room, tiptoeing around the Something, he didn't need the adrenaline rush. Now, he taught young neurosurgeons, not sailors.

He taught them technical things, of course. He taught them to make incisions, to find bleeders, to anticipate, to beware of the storms that blew up, without warning, to test them.

And now he didn't need trophies, not as long as he had patients like Josh.

Josh, and the squirrels, and the hope they presented.

But he did need sailing, desperately, and it was only March.

The assistant reached down, picked up the squirrel from the operating table, and put it back in its nest of wood chips in the plastic cage. While a technician prepared the next squirrel, Tom Ducker stepped outside in the hallway to let his fingers warm up.

FOURTEEN

THE GENERAL SURGERY RESIDENT LAY SCRUNCHED UP IN A CHAIR IN A darkened office, down the hallway from the emergency room of a local hospital. The resident had been assigned to the ER for more than a month now, and his life was ruled, as never before, by a yearning for sleep. He could sleep anywhere now, even on the floor, even standing, probably, like a combat soldier. And he slept the sleep of the dead.

Suddenly the sharp snap of a light switch entered his sleeping brain, and the bright light penetrated his closed eyelids.

He scrunched up more in the chair and turned his head away from the goddamned light, but it wouldn't go away. Wake up, wake up, wake up again.

The nurse's voice cut through the sleep, and he lifted his head and blinked at the clock on the wall. It said five minutes after one. The resident thought for a second, confused. His mind responded sluggishly.

Oh. Right.

One o'clock in the morning, not one o'clock in the afternoon. Baltimore. Emergency room rotation. Yeah. Sure. All right. Okay, *I'm awake.*

He sat up and cradled his head in his hands, his mind wracked by a momentary surge of anger. He started to snap at the nurse, then stopped himself. It didn't pay to hassle the nurses. That much, at least, he had learned.

Pay attention. Another drunk?

No. The nurse didn't think so. She recited the case, quickly, hitting only the salient details. Black male, early thirties, thin. Says he can't move his right side. His wife and brother were out in the waiting room.

So, the patient wasn't alone. That meant he was important to somebody, and that told the resident something important about the patient. The problem, whatever it was, wasn't acute loneliness.

The resident was fully awake now, erect in the chair, digesting the nurse's words. The ambulance had just brought the patient in. He had collapsed at a convenience store, and he said his whole right side was numb. He was drowsy, but not too drowsy to complain about a headache.

The nurse shook her head. No. She had smelled his breath. No alcohol.

The resident's mind worked automatically, considering and cataloging. If his right side was numb, there must be something wrong with the left side of his brain.

The resident rose from the chair and stretched.

In an alcove off the nurses' station, he poured himself a cup of bitter coffee and cut it with a heaping spoonful of sugar and two packets of synthetic cream. The stuff probably caused cancer, since everything else did . . . but in the meantime it made for a clearer, less sleepy world. The fact that he would be dealing with the brain made him wary, and he wanted to be wide-awake.

When the Styrofoam cup was empty, the resident reluctantly dropped it into the trash can and walked down the hall toward the examining area, a large room behind the waiting area. Curtain partitions had been drawn around the center bed. The curtain rings squeaked as the resident pulled the fabric aside.

The man on the table turned his head slowly toward the resident. He moved his head very carefully, the care presumably commensurate with the headache.

The resident bent over the patient to reassure him. You're going to be okay, do you understand?

Richard stared coldly back at the doctor. He had used the same phony line with his own patients, and he did not find it reassuring at all.

The resident fitted the earpieces of his stethoscope into his ears and pressed the metal disk against the skin of Richard's chest. The heart sounded normal, but fast. Richard's eyes closed, and he seemed to drift off.

Absently, the doctor pulled the stethoscope off, folded it once, and stuffed it into the pocket of his wrinkled white jacket. Suppressing a yawn, he reached for the chart and opened it.

The record said Richard was a counselor, or something, at one of the local psychiatric treatment centers. Ex-alcoholics, ex-addicts and ex-schizophrenics often worked at such places.

The resident's eyes automatically scanned the insides of Richard's arms. No needle tracks.

Whenever the brain is involved, drugs and alcohol must always be considered. Even if the patient is seriously ill with something unrelated to drug use, addiction can seriously complicate the diagnosis.

So could insanity.

The brain is perfectly capable of ordering one half of itself to stop working. Hysteria, as it's called, can mimic other diseases, including stroke.

The resident was of the opinion that hysteria was a lot more common than was reported.

On the other hand, when you couldn't figure out what was the matter, it was seductively easy to write it off as hysteria. And that was a cop-out, a potentially deadly one.

He walked back to the bedside.

Richard?

No answer. The brain, like the kidney, loses function when it is sick. When the kidney's seriously ill, urine output drops. When the brain's sick, consciousness ebbs.

Richard!

Slowly, Richard opened his eyes.

Quickly, unobtrusively, the resident put his face close enough to the patient's to check the nurse's estimate of his sobriety.

Nope. The nurse was correct. The drowsiness wasn't alcohol. The drowsiness wasn't deep enough to lessen the man's sensitivity to pain, either. His head hurt, Richard said. He asked for something to stop the pain.

Sure, the resident lied. In a little bit. When I get through. In fact the resident had no intention of giving Richard anything for his headache. As long as he could feel the pain through the drowsiness, the drowsiness wasn't getting worse. As long as Richard was complaining, he was alive.

Tell me, the resident demanded, tell me exactly where it hurts.

It hurts in my back, it feels like somebody hit me.

Did they?

No. I was in a car, and my right leg wouldn't work, and now I can't move my side. Please give me something for the headache.

The resident laid two fingers in the palm of Richard's hand. I'll give you something in a little bit. Squeeze my fingers.

Where are you, Richard?

What's the date?

Who is the president?

Did you fall?

Have you been taking anything, any drugs?

The resident went through the entire litany, but discovered nothing new. He finally turned away, walked over to the counter, opened a cupboard door and looked, frowning, for the ophthalmoscope.

It wasn't in its usual place. He stood at the cupboard for a moment, resenting the aggravations of residency.

The corollary to Murphy's Law is that if a tool is where it's supposed to be, it's broken. Otherwise, somebody would have borrowed it.

Maybe whoever borrowed the ophthalmoscope brought it back, but put it in the wrong place.

The resident muttered to himself. The advantage of rotating through the emergency room was that you learned to do without all sorts of absolutely necessary stuff. You learned to take care of the patient under the worst of circumstances. If he couldn't find the ophthalmoscope, he would simply do without it.

He was already pretty sure this fellow, what's-his-name, Richard, wouldn't be staying here, at this hospital. If he had something wrong with his brain, then he didn't belong here. If he was stroked out, he'd have to go over to University for the neuro residents to worry about him.

Presumably something in this fellow's head had cut loose for some reason and started bleeding. Maybe it was still bleeding, and if Richard got any drowsier, the resident would work faster. Far better that Richard should die in the hands of the neuro boys. Especially at this godawful hour of the night.

The resident would be very surprised if Richard didn't have a plumbing problem of some sort, a vessel that was clogged, or broken.

The arteries ran through the brain like high-pressure hoses, throbbing in syncopation with the heartbeats far below, in the chest. The big vessels branched and branched again. Blood flowed from the high-pressure arteries to the low-pressure veins, passing glucose and oxygen to the gray jelly as it passed.

The gray jelly, of course, was under almost no pressure at all.

The system was a highly efficient one, but far from foolproof. As the arteries aged and atherosclerosis began to alter them, a chunk of tissue or a blood clot could break off and be carried upward, finally lodging where an artery forked and grew smaller. Six minutes later, a piece of brain suffocated. But that usually happened in older patients. Richard was a little young for an occlusive stroke.

In someone Richard's age, it was more likely to be a hemorrhagic stroke, a bleed. Perhaps an aneurysm.

An aneurysm developed at a weak spot in an arterial wall. Over the months and years, the weak arterial wall bulged outward under the relentless, pounding pressure. An aneurysm could grow to the size of a pea, and even larger, before it ruptured.

When a vessel ruptures, the blood erupts out into the brain, ripping away connections, battering neurons, like a fire hose directed against the finest and most delicate computer anywhere. The rising tide of blood quickly finds a path to the spinal canals and, mixing with the spinal fluid, rises into the high ventricles. All over the brain, pressure rises. The process can take a few minutes, or it can be quick, like getting hit in the head with a hammer.

As he thought about his patient, the resident rummaged through the cabinet drawers, looking for the ophthalmoscope. In a moment, if he didn't find it, he'd go scrounge a penlight.

He should probably carry one, but, on the other hand, he should probably carry everything. New residents always try. You can always tell a new resident; he rattles when he walks.

Of course, Richard could also bleed through a rupture in an arteriovenous malformation, an AVM. That was basically a birth defect, something that started out as a tiny opening from an artery directly into a network of veins. The blood squirted in under high pressure, and the vein, while not very strong, was strong enough to contain the flow. For a decade or two, no one would know anything was wrong.

But as the years passed, the thin veins would balloon outward under the high-pressure blood from the arteries. In this respect an AVM was very much like an aneurysm, but an AVM could grow large.

By the time an AVM victim was Richard's age, the unsuspected tangle of overstretched veins might have grown to the size of a walnut. Then, inevitably, as the veins enlarged and were stretched thinner and thinner, a pinhole leak would develop.

The powerful spray of blood would sweep across the delicate neurons, battering at connections, ripping off boutons, sending the pressure up throughout the skull.

Either way, if it was a bleed, Richard would probably end up on the neurosurgery ward. The resident didn't envy him.

The young doctor continued to rummage through the cabinet. Suddenly, he stopped, staring in surprise at the black instrument box.

The ophthalmoscope! He had been ready to give up.

Triumphantly, he removed the box from the drawer, set it on the counter, opened it, took out the instrument and touched its switch. The tight beam of light focused on his hand.

Wow. The batteries even worked.

He walked over to the patient.

Richard?

Richard, look at the ceiling.

Groggily, Richard obeyed.

The resident focused the light first in the right eye, and then in the left. Both pupils contracted quickly. Whatever was going on in Richard's head, the lizard brain was still functioning.

The resident squinted through the back of the instrument, down the beam of light, toward Richard's retina. He found the papilla, where the optic nerve joined the eye, and it appeared normal. Perhaps the pressure in the skull hadn't been elevated long enough for the optic nerve to become inflamed.

The resident stood up and thought.

All the evidence was consistent with a bleed. But it was also consistent with hysteria—or malingering. If he sent a malingerer to University, he wouldn't hear the last of it for weeks.

Richard? Richard! Squeeze my fingers. Richard, pay attention. Don't go to sleep, Richard! Your neck hurts? Okay. I'll give you something in a minute.

An aching neck was symptomatic of a bleed. Bloody meningitis, the textbooks called it. It's an inflammation caused by blood getting loose in the brain.

Blood is not an inert substance. It's a substitute for the ancient sea that once fed man's single-celled ancestors, a sea now enclosed in vessels, converted to an all-purpose cafeteria, roadway and sewer. Waste-processing structures in the kidneys and intestines keep the flow of chemical garbage to a so-so minimum, and that's fine for most of the body's cells.

Not so the finicky neuron. To protect the neuron from the garbage in the bloodstream, nature altered the cells that line the tiniest vessels, the capillaries.

Elsewhere in the body the capillary cells are very loosely connected to one another, and substances can pass freely into and out of the vessels. But in the brain, the capillary cells join more tightly to form a fine sieve. Small molecules, like oxygen and glucose, can get through. Larger things, like garbage, bacteria and viruses, can't.

When a vessel ruptures and blood seeps through the brain, the organ suffers an allergic reaction and the cells begin to swell. The brain itself doesn't hurt, since it has no nerves, but the delicate membranes can cause excruciating pain.

That was probably what was happening to Richard, assuming, always, that he wasn't simply a hysteric.

Was the paralysis real?

The resident looked reflectively at the young man lying on the metal table. In the practical world of the emergency room, panic could be a useful diagnostic tool. The doctor stepped to the table, grabbed its left edge and tipped it.

Richard's eyes snapped open in fright as he felt himself beginning to slide. His left hand grabbed convulsively for a support.

But, as the resident observed, his right hand didn't move at all. The resident let go of the table and stepped back. Richard glared at him, angrily. Now the resident was convinced.

If Richard could have moved his right hand, he damned well would have. He still might be a hysteric, but he wasn't faking it.

The resident put the ophthalmoscope back in its box, opened the patient record, and wrote a note. There was a rush, now. If Richard died here, there would be a lot of explaining to do.

When he finished writing, the resident left the cubicle and called the hospital operator. He yawned while she activated the chief resident's beeper.

The senior man sounded sleepy when he finally phoned. The conversation was terse, with a minimum of pleasantries.

The emergency room resident listed Richard's symptoms.

No, he's not drunk, no evidence of drug use. Pupils normal, but he's paralyzed on his right side. He's drowsy and he complains of headache and a stiff neck. It sounds like he's had an intracranial bleed somewhere in the left hemisphere.

Yes, the senior man agreed. Transfer him.

The next telephone call was to the neurosurgical resident on duty at the University of Maryland Hospital. The next one was to the city ambulance service.

Less than an hour after Richard's arrival, the resident went into the waiting room to meet the patient's wife and brother. Uncomfortably, the resident explained that Richard had probably had a stroke or a cerebral hemorrhage, and that he needed to be transferred right away to University Hospital.

He made the conversation as brief as he could, and then went back to the office. But there was no sleeping, now.

It bothered him, somehow, that the man's wife was pregnant. She had appeared very frightened, and he hadn't been able to say much to reassure her. He wondered what she would do, how she would live, and what would happen to the child.

And he was grateful for the decision he had made, years ago now, to have nothing at all to do with neurology or neurosurgery. They were interesting specialties, true enough, but they were depressing as hell.

FIFTEEN

THERE IS A GRAPEVINE MAINTAINED BY PEOPLE WITH DESPERATE DISEASES, and by people who love those people. They send one another newspaper clippings and advice, and provide understanding.

There's a brain surgeon at the University of Maryland who doesn't give up on glioblastoma multiforme, the grapevine said. His name is Michael Salcman.

They came to the University of Maryland to find this doctor, and the doctor was not hard to find. The grapevine rumor was right. He didn't turn them away.

Not turning them away was not the same thing as helping them, however. Searching for ideas, Dr. Salcman began collecting papers on the disease and reading them at night, or between operations.

There really wasn't very much in the literature, which wasn't surprising. Who would want to write a paper about such a depressing disease? As a result, glioblastoma multiforme's depressing qualities were closely matched by its aura of mystery.

It was cancer, but that really didn't tell a scientist much. Cancer was a lot of things.

Some cancers behaved like a wart whose cells somehow seeded throughout the body, spreading, with new growths sprouting at large distances from the primary one: *Metastasis*, the process was called.

The popular theory was that cancers seeded by sloughing off cells that were carried along in the bloodstream until they lodged somewhere, took root, and grew secondary tumors. That's why removing a lung cancer tumor didn't cure the patient. Lung cancers seeded while they were very small, and by the time they showed up on the X-ray there were already thriving new tumors in, say, the liver.

Glioblastoma multiforme was peculiar in that it never spread outside the central nervous system. But within the skull it metastasized rapidly. Perhaps the tumor cells moved throughout the body like any other cancer, but could only survive in the brain.

Or perhaps the tumor invaded by growing microscopic tentacles that extended out into the rest of the brain. Or perhaps it spread like a plague, a microscopic disease process that marched across the landscape of living cells.

Or maybe it was something different yet. Maybe a brain cancer patient simply had brain cancer, everywhere in the brain, in the genes of every cell. In that case the tumor was just a symptom, as red splotches are a symptom of the measles. That could explain why you couldn't cure glioblastoma multiforme by cutting it out. You couldn't cure the measles by removing the spots, either.

Whatever the mechanism of its spread, glioblastoma multiforme could not be surgically contained. The visible tumor could be removed but it would come back, growing even faster, in adjacent areas of the brain. It would continue to grow, unabated, regardless of surgery, relentlessly converting the healthy tissue into a grotesque, swollen parody of itself. In the end, the patient died.

Dr. Salcman didn't know what made a glial cell turn into glioblastoma multiforme, and he didn't expect the scientific papers to tell him. But he had hoped to find *something* in the literature that would help him help his patients.

Instead, he read again and again that glioblastoma multiforme had all the worst attributes of all the worst malignant diseases. It struck people in the prime of life, grew rapidly, responded to nothing, and killed without exception.

Patients with suspected brain cancers were treated, the literature said, in a standard way. An operation was scheduled, and the neurosurgeon opened the patient's head. As soon as the surgeon reached the tumor, he snipped off a little piece and sent it to pathology.

If the growth was cancerous but the star-shaped astrocytes still looked pretty much like healthy servant cells, the pathologist would tell the surgeon it was a "grade-one astrocytoma." That was good news, as such things go.

It told the surgeon that if he painstakingly removed all the tumor he could see, his patient would have some time. Time to finish college, have a baby, write a book.

If the astrocytes were a little more deformed, the microscopic landscape a little more tortured, it was a "grade-two astrocytoma." That gave the patient time, say, for an around-the-world cruise—or to learn to fly.

A "grade-three" left him with a fishing trip or a flight to Vegas with money he didn't need any more. Dr. Salcman knew one man who had gone to the Canadian woods for the moose hunt he'd always dreamed of.

But if the microscopic landscape was tortured beyond recognition, if the cells were so malformed the pathologist could barely identify them as astrocytes, then the situation changed drastically. Under the microscope, glioblastoma cells weren't just astrocytes gone crazy. Everything appeared changed, even the blood vessels.

Technically, such a tumor might be called a "grade-four astrocytoma." There was once a movement among purists to call it that.

But "glioblastoma multiforme," according to *Pathologic Basis of Disease*, is a name that fits, a name that "makes the lesion sound as impressive and as important as it really is."

Calling glioblastoma multiforme a "grade-four astrocytoma" was like calling a hangman a "rope technician." Glioblastoma it had always been, and glioblastoma it remained.

Glioblastoma multiforme meant long-distance telephone calls, a will, maybe an early Christmas.

As Dr. Salcman read the scientific literature, he was struck by the magnitude of medicine's failure with the disease. At one time or another, neurosurgeons had tried almost everything on glioblastoma multiforme, but the mortality rate remained one hundred percent.

The disease usually wasn't even diagnosed until late in its course. The patient came in when the tumor had squeezed a spinal fluid channel shut, causing intracranial pressure to rise and consciousness to drop —or when the growth was pressing on something that caused headaches or double vision.

It usually helped to operate, to scoop out all the tumor that could be seen. The hole that remained in the brain relieved the pressure, temporarily, until the glioblastoma multiforme grew back and filled it. The patient usually survived for about six months.

There was always the nagging question, of course: Had the neurosurgeon really removed all of the tumor? Perhaps it grew back because some of it had been left in the brain.

It is truly difficult to remove all of a tumor from the brain. If the surgeon goes a millimeter too far, what remains of his patient's life will be lived as a cripple. So neurosurgeons tend to be conservative.

Still, Dr. Salcman read reports of glioblastoma multiforme tumors that had been discovered small, and that grew far forward in the uncritical prefrontal lobe. The surgeons could, and did, take out the whole lobe. They got the tumor and several centimeters of healthy tissue behind it.

It seemed to make little difference. Such patients died about six months later of recurrent tumor.

Surgeons had tried operating a second time, when the tumor recurred, but the patients usually didn't . . . do well.

This, Dr. Salcman thought, might be a result of technical problems. The scarring from the first operation tended to obscure the landmarks, which made it more likely that the surgeon would discover an artery the hard way or touch something connected to the patient's ability to hear, see, or move.

Even if the second operation was technically successful, the time gained was negligible. Glioblastoma multiforme tumors, as time passed, grew faster.

The problem had been confronted by other doctors. One of the more notable efforts had been launched by the Baltimore branch of the National Cancer Institute, which occupied the ninth floor of the University of Maryland Hospital.

The cancer research center had money, talent, and a record of success—doctors there had been instrumental in developing the cure for Hodgkin's disease, a cancer of the lymph nodes. Hodgkin's disease, when the center began to study it, had been as relentless and deadly as glioblastoma multiforme.

The center attempted to treat patients with glioblastoma multiforme, using every technique known. Doctors tried the new chemical therapies that were proving so promising for other malignancies, like breast cancer. But the blood-brain barrier prevented those drugs from reaching the brain tumor cells, and the result was nil.

Finally the specialists concluded that glioblastoma multiforme was simply untreatable, and they quit accepting patients who had it.

That deeply troubled Dr. Ducker, who thought that somebody ought to at least try to help those patients. The result was that his second-in-command became a glioblastoma multiforme expert.

Having no choice, Dr. Salcman agreed to do his best, and his best could be very good indeed. He accepted the patients, he operated on them, and he watched them all die.

As patient after patient came to him, and appealed for help, and as he failed them, it became increasingly difficult for him to remember that the disease was an unconscious process, a mindless dance of molecules, a formless, shapeless Something. As his patients died, one by one, a frustration built and turned to anger. He grew to hate glioblastoma multiforme.

Inevitably, in the mind of the surgeon as in the minds of his patients, an impossible hope grew. No one had ever been cured, but might not there be a first?

Michael Salcman would wage war on glioblastoma. If it was the perfect killing machine, then it was also the perfect enemy, the perfect challenge.

Glioblastoma multiforme was a relatively rare disease, one that struck perhaps ten thousand Americans a year. That meant that it was somewhat less common than Hodgkin's disease, and occurred perhaps one tenth as frequently as lung cancer. But a lot of doctors treated those more common illnesses, and almost no one specialized in glioblastoma multiforme. As soon as glioblastoma multiforme patients heard about Dr. Salcman, the disease became a common ailment on the twelfth floor of University Hospital.

Dr. Salcman's patients were almost always those who had been given up on by other surgeons. The patients had almost all had one operation, followed by a maximum dose of radiation, followed by chemotherapy. Then the tumor had recurred, and their doctors had counseled them to accept the inevitable.

Many patients accepted that advice, and perhaps wisely so. Dr. Salcman didn't see them, however. He saw only the fighters. They looked at him and said, "Doc, I'm going to lick this thing."

Dr. Salcman said he would try, but . . .

The patient vowed to be brave, and not complain, and be a model patient.

. . . but, Dr. Salcman said, there would be some trade-offs.

When he saw their X-rays and CAT scans, he understood why their original surgeon had given up. The first operation had left a big hole, and the tumor had grown back in, filling that space, and had continued to expand. In a second operation, more of the brain would have to be taken.

There was a risk, always a risk.

Anything, doc. Please.

Dr. Salcman explained that he would go in after the tumor again, but he wanted the patient to understand that there were no capsules around glioblastoma multiforme tumors. It would be difficult to tell where the tumor ended and, say, vision began.

Under the very best of circumstances, every brain was different. There were no little signposts to mark the motor cortex, where movement originates. There were no landmarks defining the speech area. There were no red lights flashing, saying, "Beware, this is Wernicke's area and if you enter, the patient will never again understand what another human being says to him."

With the skull jammed with scar tissue and overgrown tumor, the brain topography would be gnarled and changed. It would be easy for the surgeon to touch something that was attached to something . . .

Dr. Salcman studied the CAT scans, and wondered. Perhaps the first surgeon had been right to give up. The trouble was, Michael Salcman didn't have that option.

If he was going to do second operations on glioblastoma multiforme, a procedure that the literature said didn't work, Dr. Salcman would have to do something different enough to justify some scrap of hope, for himself as well as for his patients. And yet, he could think of nothing new to do.

Then . . . maybe he should just do it *better*.

Without hope, you didn't do your best work. In that way, perhaps, Dr. Salcman could be different. Whereas earlier surgeons had used their naked eye and the suction device to pick away the glioblastoma multiforme tissue, Dr. Salcman worked under an operating microscope, vaporizing the tumor with a laser beam. In Dr. Salcman's view the laser was one of the most important advances in neurosurgery since Cushing's day. It allowed the surgeon to fulfill the old, previously impossible imperative. With the laser, you could operate on the brain without touching it.

Yes, he told his patients, he thought he might be able to extend their lives. He couldn't cure them, but he'd see them again when the tumor came back. By then, he might have something else worth trying.

Dr. Salcman was careful to look directly at the patient. "There is a chance I can help, but you must be prepared to trade. You may have to give me your left arm so that I can get more of the tumor out. I may make your speech worse. One side of your body may be paralyzed."

He tried to inform them, but at the same time he attempted not to burden them with his private nightmares.

"If you cut a leg off, your patient is still the same human being," he once reflected. "If you remove a man's arm, he's still the same human being. But if something goes wrong in a brain operation on Uncle Charlie, he may no longer be Uncle Charlie.

"He is no longer the person everybody knew and loved. He no longer understands what you say to him. He no longer moves around. One side of his face sags or droops. There is nothing subtle about a neurosurgical disaster."

But it was a risk he knew he would have to take.

He waited in his office while the families stepped outside to talk it over.

They really had no choice. To say no was to die. To say yes was to die, too, except, maybe, a miracle . . . and that was hope. The families talked it over, but they didn't come to Baltimore from Seattle, or Maine, or Oklahoma, just to give up. They usually reached a decision quickly.

Michael Salcman could give them hope but, in the end, he had no miracles.

In return for the hope, each patient gave Dr. Salcman one gift. Each one gave the neurosurgeon another chance to observe the enemy up close.

What he saw was grim.

Glioblastoma multiforme invaded everything it touched. Saddest of all, the tumor had an affinity for the corpus callosum, the bridge of tissue between the left and right sides of the brain. Too often it traveled across that bridge, invading both frontal lobes, with hideous consequences.

It is those big frontal lobes that distinguish the brains of men from those of monkeys. While their role is diffuse—one of the two can be completely removed without disturbing the personality—the functioning of at least one lobe is absolutely necessary. If both are destroyed, the personality loses something indefinable.

When Dr. Salcman saw that the patient was lethargic, distant, and indifferent to his fate, he knew it was too late. The tumor had crossed the corpus callosum, destroyed both frontal lobes and effectively given the patient a lobotomy. The CAT scan usually confirmed the guess: tumor in both lobes. Hopeless.

But whenever he could find a measure of hope, a hope of a little more useful life for a patient, he fought with every skill and tool at his command. Using the microscope, he directed the laser at the tumor, carefully, carefully, burning it out of every nook and cranny, trying to remove it all, as though there were something to win, as though the patient might be saved.

It was a fiction, of course, because the patients always died. But as the months passed, the statistics showed a definite increase in the length of time the patients survived.

As with Cushing's first patients, some of them eked out another year of useful life. And that, for glioblastoma multiforme patients, was notable.

Dr. Salcman still couldn't cure glioblastoma patients, but as the survival figures were confirmed again and again, he became convinced that he was headed in the right direction.

If a glioblastoma multiforme patient could live a year, why not eighteen months? If he could live eighteen months, why not two years? If two years . . . ?

Still, if he were going to achieve longer and longer survival times, Dr. Salcman suspected he would have to use more than just surgery. For one thing, by the time a patient got to him there was a finite limit on how much brain he had left to lose. Dr. Salcman could hardly remove any more. And there didn't seem any way, any way at all, that he could ever remove every last cancer cell in surgery.

It had taken combination treatments of surgery, radiation, and chemotherapy to cure leukemia and Hodgkin's disease. If anything, glioblastoma multiforme was more resistant than those.

But they couldn't take any more radiation. By the time a patient got to Dr. Salcman, he had had so much radiation that the skin on his scalp was like leather, and almost refused to heal. Any more radiation and something was sure to go wrong.

Chemical therapy, then, seemed the only way for him to kill the cancer cells that remained after surgery. But the blood-brain barrier kept the drugs from getting to the tumor.

Dr. Salcman wondered whether drugs couldn't be found to open up the blood-brain barrier long enough to let the cancer-killing drugs through. There were chemicals that, in theory, ought to do that. They had been tried before, though not with much success. Perhaps, if Michael Salcman just tried a little harder . . .

The experiments were done whenever Dr. Salcman had the time and when the CAT-scanner was free. He would put a dog in a scanner, inject what he hoped would be a barrier-opening drug, and then quickly follow it with a marker chemical. Then the dog's head would be scanned, to see if any of the marker got into the brain.

It didn't. So he tried a different technique. Nothing really worked, but he kept trying. He couldn't think of anything better to do. He tried again, and again, and again. And still it didn't work, and his patients died.

Meanwhile, Dr. Salcman had to find time to teach and to treat various employees of the big University of Maryland medical complex. He liked to teach, and he didn't mind at all treating the employees. They almost never had glioblastoma multiforme, and they rarely died.

There was Dr. George Samaras, for instance. He was a bioengineer from radiation therapy. His shoulder was killing him.

Dr. Salcman examined him, and disagreed. It wasn't his shoulder that hurt, though it felt like it. There was a compressed nerve in the neck, and when it was pinched it sent ouch messages to the brain. The brain thought the messages were coming from the shoulder, but the brain was wrong.

He might need a disc operation on his neck, to relieve the pressure. Michael put the bioengineer in the hospital and scheduled tests.

Until then, the neurosurgeon really hadn't known Dr. Samaras. They had nodded in the hallways but they had never had a conversation or drunk a beer together. But as Dr. Samaras lived for a few days on the neurosurgical floor, the two got to talking shop. That meant research.

Dr. Samaras was studying cancer, too, it turned out. He was attempting to capitalize on one of cancer's most puzzling peculiarities, its sensitivity to heat. For some poorly understood reason, when cancer cells were heated they often became very vulnerable to drugs and, even, to the body's own defense mechanisms.

Some lung cancer patients recovered spontaneously when they got pneumonia and developed high fevers. Scientists had theorized that it was the burning fevers that did, well, whatever.

Dr. Samaras was involved in building microwave antennas for heating tissue.

It hadn't worked so far, but Dr. Samaras thought that might be because of the way the heat was being applied. Heat behaved in a certain way as it passed through tissue, and tended to dissipate rapidly. Theoretically, the cancer most vulnerable to heat would be a round one, sort of . . .

A round one?

Glioblastoma multiforme was a generally round growth. Suddenly, Dr. Salcman was very, very interested.

He had never paid a lot of attention to heat therapy, but as Dr. Samaras talked, the idea sounded better and better. Theoretically, it might make sense. Normal brain cells were exquisitely sensitive to high temperatures. That might imply that cancerous ones would be even more vulnerable.

Could they rig up a set of microwave antennas around the patient's head, adjusted so that the beams would converge inside the skull, precisely where the tumor was?

They prepared a research request and sent it to the National Institutes of Health. The people at NIH thought it sounded like a good idea, and agreed to finance it.

But the two scientists found out rather quickly that the idea, like all others that had been tried on glioblastoma multiforme, was not very useful. Microwaves didn't penetrate flesh very well. Their early experiments revealed that, in order to heat the interior of the brain, the microwave beams would have to be strong enough to roast the scalp and skull.

The two scientists set about rethinking their approach. Perhaps it would be better to insert an antenna inside the head, in the hole left after tumor removal.

Dr. Samaras knew of a suitable antenna that had been constructed for other uses. The scientist who designed and built it was a Dr. Leonard Taylor, on the university's College Park campus.

That posed another problem. Putting an antenna outside of the head, where it could be tinkered with, was one thing. Putting one inside of the skull was quite a different matter. What would happen if it didn't get hot enough? There was some indication in the literature that the glioblastoma multiforme cells, if heated just slightly, would grow faster.

For that matter, with the brain itself so sensitive to heat, what would happen if the antenna got too hot?

The microwave generator, which controlled the power that went to the antenna inside the head, would have to be very carefully constructed, very carefully indeed. For something so important, the two men would have preferred to get the support of some big electronics company, with a team of experts. Unfortunately, there wasn't anywhere near that much money left in their research grant.

As a result, the first experimental microwave generator was, well . . . custom-built. A scientist who can't lay his hands on the odd transistor or cathode-ray tube will sooner or later end up teaching freshmen at a cow college. The machine grew from wire, solder, scavenged and borrowed parts, determination and long, long hours.

Again and again, they went from the drawing board to the animal lab. Months passed and the contraption evolved, growing steadily safer, easier to sterilize, and more reliable.

Finally, it was time to try it.

It was easy to find a patient.

The first use of the device was a sensation in the hospital, and the public relations office sent out a press release. The story of the doc who put a microwave antenna in people's heads got the instant attention of editors. Various reports appeared in local papers, and versions of those moved on the national wire services.

The reporters all asked, "Did it work?"

Dr. Salcman patiently explained that he didn't really know. What he did know was that the first patient, a German businessman, had sur-

vived the heating without side effects. That helped to address what
had to be the first question, which was safety.

What would happen now was problematical.

So the reporters couldn't say it worked, but they talked to the patients and found that they had a story anyway. The story was that the
University of Maryland team was trying something new against the
deadliest brain cancer of all. That, in itself, was news.

Glioblastoma is a rare disease, but the United States is a large country.

The stories got clipped out of newspapers and mailed to friends and
relatives with brain tumors. Hundreds of dying people, looking for
something to try, anything, resolved to put their faith in the doctor
from Baltimore.

The long-distance calls came in from housewives, parents, children.

Dr. Salcman was swamped.

He had only one empty moment left in his life, and that was noon-
time. He instructed his secretary, Sharon Wellslager, to take messages
and arrange them each morning on his desk.

Then, as he ate, he could go through the pleas and return telephone
calls. It was a very efficient routine, and a necessary one. But it made
lunch very, very depressing.

CHAPTER
SIXTEEN

JOE? THE JUNIOR RESIDENT SAID, LOUDLY.

Joe?

Joe Trott's lips moved and the resident bent low over the bed.

Good. If the boy responded to his name, he knew who he was. A majority of neurons had to be operating before a brain knew its name.

The surgical intensive care unit was on the seventh floor of the old Halsted building at the Hopkins, very close to the surgical suites. The sign on the door said SICU but the staff pronounced it Sick-U. You had to be very sick to be in the Sick-U.

It had been after dark by the time Joe arrived in the SICU cubicle. A neurosurgical nurse stood by, waiting for him. As soon as his bed lurched to a stop, she started working down her checklist, attaching the tubes and monitors that would help her keep him alive.

As for the resident, the first thing he had to do was find out just how sick Joe really was. For a moment he stood thoughtfully over the bed. His right hand absently touched the safety pin in his lapel.

The pin was a tool as well as a badge of office. If people are working properly, they react when you stick them with a pin. If they don't react, something is definitely wrong.

Not that any self-respecting neurosurgeon would ever "stick a patient with a pin." The pin was used to "apply a painful stimulus."

The resident's fingers dropped from his lapel, reached into the right pocket of his coat, and wrapped around the penlight.

Joe? the resident asked, again.

The boy was groggy. That was understandable.

JOE?

A little louder.

JOE?

Hearing is a primitive system, which makes it one of the first to recover after surgery. But sometimes you had to yell.

Joe!

Joe's eyelids fluttered.

Joe, you're in the intensive care unit. The operation is over and you're fine.

Nobody was fine in the SICU—that would be a contradiction. But reassurance was part of the medicine. Besides, the resident would feel silly yelling something like, hey, fellow, you're as close to death as you'll ever be, and you may be stupid or paralyzed, we can't tell yet. Bedside etiquette demanded a reassurance.

The resident flicked on the penlight. The tiny beam reflected off the stainless-steel bed railing.

Joe! Look at the ceiling, Joe.

Slowly, Joe looked up.

Good. He was responding.

The resident directed the light beam through the lens of Joe's right eye. As the light touched the retina, the stimulation raced back into the brain, following the optic nerves to the back of the head and then echoing through all three brains. Almost instantly the brains responded and the pupil contracted.

The process involved all levels of the brain. If something went wrong, somewhere, the first symptom would often be a slow pupil response. Joe's pupils contracted with satisfying speed, and the resident put the penlight back in his pocket.

The resident was never without his penlight, and the more nervous he was, the more often he reached for it. This early in his residency, the young doctor used it almost constantly. Working in the SICU made him very nervous. It was supposed to.

Sometimes it seemed that everything was expected of a second-year neurosurgical resident. He examined patients, filled out forms, ordered medicine, watched surgery, answered the beeper, ordered laboratory studies . . . and got to go home every other night, and one weekend in three, assuming he wasn't busy in the lab.

A few years ago, one of the Hopkins residents gave up his apartment and moved his clothes to the hospital. Why pay rent? He never got to go home.

But someday it will all pay off. He'll be a board-certified brain surgeon. He won't carry a beeper because he'll have residents to do it for him, and he'll have the power to cut into the brain of a human being, carefully, carefully, and tie an aneurysm or remove a piece of flesh, and restore a life.

The resident opened up Joe's curled hand and laid two fingers across the palm.

Joe! Squeeze my fingers, Joe.

Slowly, painfully, the hand closed around the fingers, but there was no strength there. That wasn't remarkable, considering how long Dr. Murray and Dr. Long had puttered around in his posterior fossa. The resident had gone in and watched for a while. It was remarkable that the kid was alive at all, considering the size of the tumor.

Joe! Wiggle your toes, Joe.

Joe!

Slowly, Joe's right big toe wiggled, then, after a moment, his left.

Thoughtfully, the resident picked up Joe's patient record and walked out to the nurses' station. There was an empty chair there, but he didn't take it. He was too tired, and if he sat down he'd relax. Right now he needed to be alert, so he stood at the counter and wrote his assessment.

If the resident hadn't wanted to be a neurosurgeon so badly, he could have been a general surgeon much more easily. In just two more years he could have gone out to a community hospital to do hernias and gall bladders and make payments on a medium-large house. He still could. It wasn't too late.

But what was a gall bladder? A gall bladder was the organ of bile. The brain was the organ of personality! It took nine years of training before they'd give you a license to touch it.

For the moment, there was work to do, a night to survive, then another day. He rested the clipboard on the formica counter and started writing the drug orders.

The first prescription was for steroids, the closest thing neurosurgery had to a wonder drug. Steroids could control swelling. Unfortunately, steroids knocked down the patient's immune system, and infection was a worry, anyway, after surgery.

On the other hand, if Joe's brain was swelling and cutting off its own circulation, and the resident didn't give him steroids, the boy wouldn't live to get an infection.

Another side effect was that steroids sometimes made people a little crazy. That could be a problem. Sometimes, when you put a sick and frightened patient on steroids, you also had to tie him down.

As for infection, the next prescription was for eight thousand milligrams of antibiotic a day. Joe had been open for a long, long time in the operating room.

Back in the early days of neurosurgery, patients often died in the operating room. The surgeon touched something that was connected to something that was connected to something, or something unexpected happened and he met Big Red. Now, with eighty years of tradition, and the operating microscope, patients rarely died on the table.

That didn't mean they didn't die. They just didn't die on the table. They died in SICU, and one of the chief things they died of was infection. Ordering the antibiotic would make everyone feel more comfortable.

Then the resident wrote a prescription for a stool softener (he certainly didn't want the patient straining), and then another for a stomach antacid. The nurse could give him Tylenol suppositories and codeine injections for pain.

The resident stood there a moment and worried. They used to die on the operating table, but they didn't any more. If they died now they died in the SICU. Of brain swelling. Of hemorrhage. Of infection. Of something.

As an afterthought, the resident wrote a prescription for a vitamin tablet. He snapped Joe's record shut, returned to the cubicle and briefly stood by the bed, checking the monitors. Automatically, he noted the bilious liquid in the bottle on the floor. It had collected there after draining from Joe's stomach via a long tube that entered the boy's right nostril and ran down his throat. The fluid was pretty ghastly. The antacid should help.

The worry, there, was a stress ulcer. Rats develop ulcers if you torture them. If you take people and cut holes in their heads, and poke around near their brain stems, their stomachs tend to respond the same way.

At the other end of Joe's metabolism, a soft Foley catheter disappeared into his penis. It carried urine directly from the bladder to a sterile plastic container with graduated volume markings on it.

The resident would have to watch closely for signs of a bladder infection. A bladder infection was one of the many things that could kill a post-op brain surgery patient.

Still another tube, this one of thin plastic, protruded from beneath the turban of bandages on Joe's head. One end was attached to the catheter that the surgeons had left in a ventricle. Through the catheter they could continue to measure intracranial pressure and, if necessary, it would allow them to drain off cerebrospinal fluid and relieve the pressure.

There was the usual trade-off. Pressure readings from inside the head could allow the doctors to monitor brain swelling and fine-tune the therapy. On the other hand, bacteria could climb up the tube and enter the brain. The tube, like everything else, would have to be handled carefully.

The nurses would keep watch throughout the night, and every fifteen minutes they would record the readings. If anything changed, well . . . a nurse was one of the many people who had the power to make the resident's beeper go off. Someone once computed that the average second-year resident gets between one and three hours of sleep on his duty nights.

Joe's resident could sleep sitting up in a chair, and he knew the precise location of every couch in the area. Sometimes there was even an empty bed, and that was heaven. But wherever he was, the beeper was with him.

To the resident's relief, Joe did well as the night wore on—well, that is, considering the size and location of the hole in his head. The resident checked on him periodically throughout the next day, but the dials were always more or less where they should be.

But that evening, twenty-four hours after the operation, the beeper went off. The resident was at Joe's bedside in less than ninety seconds.

Joe had been fine during rounds. What was wrong now?

He seemed lethargic, the nurse said.

The resident reached for his penlight.

Joe?

Joe!

Squeeze my hand, Joe.

The nurse was right. Joe did seem a bit woozier, but his pupils responded well to the probing penlight. Still, the lethargy was a worry.

As the night passed, the boy's blood pressure climbed up to one hundred and eighty, at least sixty above normal, and his heart speeded up. The beeper went off again and again.

By morning Joe seemed vacant, disinterested.

Deep in the posterior fossa, something, a blood clot or injured tissue, was swelling. The swelling pinched off the supply of oxygen-laden blood and the gray cells began to suffocate. They grew sluggish, and their firing rate slowed.

Decreased circulation to the brain caused a series of complex metabolic alarms to go off. Joe's body tried, desperately, to force more oxygen-carrying blood into the head. The brain ordered the heart to accelerate, and the arteries to clamp down tighter and tighter. That drove the blood pressure up and helped the heart push blood into the skull.

Joe's resident consulted the chief resident with increasing frequency as the changes became more marked. Dr. Murray came in several times to stand by the bed and help the resident worry.

The nurse read the dials every fifteen minutes. The doctors allowed some of the spinal fluid to escape through the monitoring tube. That helped a little, but not enough.

Everybody agreed. More steroids. Steroids could make Joe a little crazy, but brain swelling could make him dead.

As the swelling continued into the second day, the rising pressure began to affect the brain stem where it narrows into the spinal cord and exits through the big hole, the foramen magnum. The brain began to lose its ability to orchestrate Joe's metabolism.

The resident worried. Joe might start losing fluids through his kidneys, or a serious disturbance might develop in his heartbeat. Or he might die without warning, as something gave way and the swelling suddenly pushed the brain stem aside.

Or he might die slowly, lethargy turning to drowsiness, drowsiness to sleep, sleep to coma, as the swelling brain pinched the arteries closed.

In one sense, the resident had little authority. He was closely watched by the chief resident, who in turn was closely watched by Dr. Murray, who was closely watched by Dr. Long, who in turn was closely watched by the ghost of Harvey Cushing.

But it was the resident who watched Joe. If the boy's heart suddenly stopped, it wouldn't be Dr. Long pumping on the chest and yelling for the defibrillator pads. It would be the resident. It had always been so.

Joe!

Hey Joe, c'mon, I know you can hear me.

Joe!

Hold up two fingers, Joe. Show me two fingers.

Two fingers twitched, trying to move.

Good. That meant he could hear, he knew who he was, he knew what a finger was, he knew what the number two was, and he could co-ordinate movements in his hand.

Death, if nearby, wasn't going to be immediate.

Joe?

Squeeze my hand, Joe.

Hey Joe, look up at the ceiling . . .

That evening, the resident helped roll Joe's bed down to the CAT-scan room. He watched from behind the leaded glass as Joe's head moved slowly, notch by notch, into the orifice of the scanner. The resident could tell that Joe was getting sleepier and sleepier by the minute. As soon as the scan was complete, the resident was back at his patient's side.

Joe!

Joe!

Wiggle your toes.

Deep in the posterior fossa, the pilot light guttered.

Joe?

Don't go to sleep!

The resident felt more comfortable when he got Joe back to the SICU. He hated to face a crisis on strange territory. When something happened, it was far better to deal with it on your home turf.

The CAT scan showed the swollen area as a dark ring around what was left of the tumor. Dr. Murray and Dr. Long examined the films and decided that tomorrow Dr. Murray would take Joe back to the operating room, reopen the surgical wound and see what was wrong and what could be done about it.

That night, the resident got to sleep in his own bed, but not for long. Early the next morning he appeared in the operating room to help get Joe ready for Dr. Murray, who would arrive about 8 A.M. As soon as the anesthetic took effect, the resident removed the bandages from the boy's head and locked his skull back into the Mayfield clamp.

In the background, the heart monitor beeped rapidly, one hundred and thirty beats a minute, as Joe's heart worked desperately to force more blood into his brain.

Dr. Murray arrived and the resident helped him open the old sutures and lay back the muscles. The unhealed incisions came apart easily. Carefully, Dr. Murray used a long pair of tweezers to lift the dura.

There was no sign of a blood clot, but the left hemisphere of the cerebellum, the organ of co-ordination, filled the view. It was swollen and angry-looking.

The heart monitor went beep-beep-beep-beep, fast but steady.

If there had been a clot, Dr. Murray could have removed it, and given the brain more space. Since there was no clot, he would have to remove a segment of the cerebellum. He normally would rather not do that, but now he had no choice. The missing tissue would provide more room for expansion, and Joe probably wouldn't notice the loss.

Carefully, gently, Dr. Murray teased apart the arachnoid membrane and the pia beneath it. Using the suction probe, he cut a trench across the bottom of the cerebellum, cutting deeper and deeper into it, coagulating the blood vessels with the bipolars. It was careful, tedious, perfectionist work, and it was an hour and a half before the severed portion of brain fell free.

When they were finished, the surgeons laid the dura back over the brain, but they didn't sew it closed. Leaving the dura unstitched would allow the brain room to bulge a little, and that might help ease the pressure.

Once again, the neck muscles were reattached to the skull and the scalp was stitched back in place with large sutures. Then the resident accompanied Joe Trott back to the SICU and Dr. Murray went to the waiting room to talk in somber tones to Joe's parents.

The anesthesiologist had administered an antidote to the anesthetic as soon as the operation ended, but when the resident got Joe back to the SICU he still seemed unconscious.

Joe?

Joe?

Squeeze my fingers!

Nothing.

The resident let the limp hand drop. In an hour, when the anesthetic had worn off completely, he'd try again.

But before he did, something happened to a little group of neurons deep in Joe's brain stem and they began to discharge their electricity all at once, aimlessly, flooding the circuits nearby. Those neurons, too, began firing rapidly. The chain reaction took only an instant to spread throughout the swollen brain.

Joe's body stiffened, and jerked violently, then jerked again. The dials swung wildly.

The resident's beeper went off.

The resident ran toward the SICU, but by the time he arrived the convulsions were over. But from the nurse's description it sounded like grand mal seizure, and that was terrifying. Convulsions raised the blood pressure even more, and heightened the risk that one of the carefully sealed bleeders inside Joe's brain could burst open.

Valium.

Valium was a relatively mild drug, and it could prevent the epileptic brain storms from beginning.

The resident injected the drug directly into the intravenous tube, then stood back for a moment. His hand groped in his pocket for the penlight. Joe's pupils responded, narrowing.

When the crisis seemed to be over the resident left, but within the hour the nurse called him back. She said Joe had been at least semiconscious until a few minutes ago. Then, without warning, he was out cold.

Joe?

There was an edge to the resident's voice.

Joe!

Nothing.

The probing beam of the penlight flashed into Joe's right eye, and the pupil reacted normally. The left eye responded as well. He was unconscious, but he wasn't dead. Not yet.

Using his thumb and forefinger, the resident found a nerve and squeezed, hard. Pain of that magnitude would reach all the way down to the lizard brain and cause the body to flinch.

But Joe didn't even twitch.

The resident and the nurse stood on either side of the bed, momentarily at a loss for what to do. A minute passed, and another.

Then, suddenly, Joe opened his eyes and looked up at them.

Joe? The resident almost shouted in relief.

Whispered: Yes.

Petit mal, the resident decided. The small seizure. A disturbance. A little thing. But near to the soul. Apparently, Valium wasn't enough to stop the seizures. Now he had to write prescriptions for two stronger anticonvulsants, Dilantin and phenobarbital. Whatever the risk, the seizures had to be controlled.

Joe?

Joe, squeeze my fingers.

Joe, what's one plus one?

Two.

Good.

Within the next few hours a second disturbing problem had developed. Joe's temperature had begun to rise. The resident conferred with the senior doctors and then ordered a more powerful antibiotic cocktail. With luck, that would take care of the infection—wherever and whatever it was.

In the meantime, the swelling problem seemed implacable. Once again, the resident accompanied Joe to the CAT-scanner. That's where the third seizure struck. Without warning, Joe quit breathing and his fingernails turned blue.

Almost in panic the resident pried open the boy's clenched teeth, forced a hard plastic airway down his throat, and helped the CAT-scan team attach the tube to the swing-arm of a respirator. Slowly, the fingernails turned pink again, but the resident didn't dare relax.

With the respirator tube in his windpipe, the boy couldn't talk—but he could move his hands.

Joe! Show me two fingers.

Weakly, the curled hand moved and two fingers stretched out.

Good. He was still conscious.

The CAT scan seemed to take forever, but there were no more seizures until Joe was back in SICU. There, Joe convulsed again and his heart raced fast, very fast, one hundred and fifty beats a minute, and some of the beats were not perfectly synchronized.

When a new dose of anticonvulsants finally took effect and the seizure ended, Joe lay exhausted on the bed, his heart rate finally diminishing. For a while he was semiconscious. Then he slept.

The resident didn't. There were no more seizures, but it was another long, watchful night. There were blood tests, and X-rays, and an updated order for anticonvulsants.

The blood study said the white count was up, which meant Joe's body was mobilizing to fight an infection. That was good, because it meant his immune system hadn't been completely stunned by the steroids. But . . .

Where was the infection?

There were no bacteria in the bladder or kidneys, because the lab said the urine was still sterile. The boy didn't have a wound infection —the resident had personally put on a new dressing just a few hours ago, and the incision hadn't been discolored or puffy. But he couldn't see the brain. If *that* was where the infection was . . .

The resident prescribed more antibiotics. Chloramphenicol and nafcillin could have some deadly side effects, but most patients could tolerate them. A brain infection had a serious side effect, too: death.

The hours passed slowly, and Joe's pilot light flickered again and again, but he didn't die.

The only hopeful sign that the resident could think of was that Joe was still there, very much there, behind the half-closed eyes. He still responded to his name, and from that, at least, the resident could draw some hope.

But from Joe's point of view, consciousness had its drawbacks.

Early one morning before the cold March dawn, as the crisis lingered and Joe lay, feverish and semiconscious, his nurse left the cubicle for a moment. Out at the nurses' station, she sent for several more vials of one of the many drugs the resident had written orders for.

Suddenly, she heard Joe cry out in anguish.

"It hurts! It hurts!"

The cry was hoarse.

The nurse stopped what she was doing, instantly. How could he cry out, with a respirator down his windpipe?

The nurse's rubber-soled shoes squeaked on the tile floor as she ran back toward the room.

Joe had ripped the respirator fitting away and pulled the gastric tube out of his nose. The turban of bandages lay on the floor. His head was white and stubbly, except for the crusted blood along the stitched-up flap. His body thrashed on the bed and he screamed in pain.

The nurse knew exactly what to do. She grabbed his flailing wrists, shouting at him through the pain, trying to prevent him from ripping out the tubes in his arms. She wrestled expertly. He was very weak, and no match for her.

There were a lot of people in the room now, holding him down and doing things. He tried to resist as they put the respirator fitting back in his windpipe, but it was no use. He was exhausted, and his mind swam under the heavy sedative.

The medical team worked quickly, wrapping loops of gauze around his wrists and ankles and tying them to the bed. They ran the gastric tube back through his nose and down his throat, readjusted the monitors, and swathed his head in fresh bandages.

And still the pain went on, and on, and on.

Joe had been right, the night before the operation, when he'd rejected the notion of running down the hallway, screaming. They'd have just grabbed him and sedated him, and it would have been all wasted energy.

It didn't pay to lose your cool.

It changed nothing.

CHAPTER
SEVENTEEN

JOE'S LIZARD BRAIN STRETCHED AGAINST THE PRESSURE, DEFORMING. THE dials jumped and the respirator sighed, and the brain cells struggled to survive.

His mind went where it would, beyond his control, and chilly mists curled through his psyche. It wasn't real, and he knew it. He knew the mists were named "morphine" or "codeine" or something like that. He knew the difference between reality and unreality, but when he was in the foggy valley, he didn't much care.

He sat on a rock and discussed the situation with Anmar.

A chain of surrealistic mountains were blue in the background, and the fog curled around Joe's feet. The valley was cold, but after a little while, Joe didn't mind. The cold made him numb, and that was better than the pain.

So it was comfortable, sitting on the rock in the foggy valley. Though he didn't see them at the moment, he knew the valley was populated with friends. When he got time, he would find Gandalf and Frodo Baggins, whom he first met in *The Lord of the Rings*. He hadn't seen Gandalf and Frodo Baggins for a long time.

But there wasn't time for that now.

The problem was that he was trapped.

He had thought they were just going to cut into his head and take the tumor out, and be done with it. He hadn't agreed to any of these experiments they were doing on him. Damn it, they were prolonging his recovery, lousing up his school schedule, yelling at him all the time, stretching out and intensifying the pain.

He had known he was going to hurt . . .

The fog grew denser, obscuring the mountains. The world contained only two beings, now. Joe Trott and Anmar.

. . . they had told him he was going to hurt, but he hadn't known they would torture him and experiment on him.

Item: There was a resident, an evil and ugly creature who, whenever he got the urge, or when it served some malevolent purpose, screamed at him and called him back from the foggy valley.

Joe always heard him coming, from far off. The man would shout his name in an impatient and demanding voice, pulling him back to the pain. Joe might be in a hell of a jam, but he wasn't stupid, and he struggled to remain in the valley.

But the resident somehow always won and the valley would clear and turn very dry, with a cracked-mud floor. Then it vanished and Joe was in the white room, under the glaring lights, and it hurt, it hurt, it hurt.

Joe!

The voice was relentless. If he didn't respond, the man would touch some place on the upper part of his leg, in a private, inside part, and find a nerve, and bring him back on a breaking wave of agony.

Anmar was imaginary, but he was a friend, and it was difficult . . . his brain was slow, from the damage they had done, and it hurt to use it. It hurt, and it required tremendous will.

The resident didn't care.

Joe!

Item: They had some kind of a torture device, a rubber tube, that they'd stuck up his nose and down the back of his throat. It was one of the ways they tied you down, and it made you feel like you were gagging all the time. You retched, but the tube wouldn't come up and the convulsive movements made your throat rub against the tube. Joe's throat hurt, terribly.

It was part of the experiments.

Item: They were holding him in a hospital room, a small one. They never turned off the lights, so the pain always had a bright, piercing quality.

It was a neat gimmick, actually. It piled psychological pain atop physical pain. Maybe the purpose of the experiment was to find the limits of endurance for people who had just had brain surgery.

The psychological torture was very real, too, and had an Oriental flavor about it. There were hard, lifeless noises, pings and clicks, beeps and gurgles, and a bell went off somewhere.

Item: He wasn't alone in his suffering. They had others trapped, too, very nearby. Occasionally he heard their anguished moans.

When Joe wasn't in the foggy valley, when he couldn't find it or when the resident pulled him back, he tried not to open his eyes. When he did open them his brain was flooded with light and information, and that overwhelmed him, made him exhausted, and then the torture was more effective. As Anmar knew, pain was worse when you were exhausted.

Joe had another reason to keep his eyes closed, at least when the doctors were around. As soon as he opened them, the doctors moved away and started whispering big, incomprehensible words to one another.

If he didn't open his eyes, they thought he was asleep and they forgot he was there. Then they would sometimes discuss the various means of torture, right by the bed. By keeping his eyes shut, Joe overheard them planning to stick some kind of needle into his brain.

The conversation jerked him right out of the valley. A needle in his brain! The thought filled Joe with dread.

"Needle . . . edema . . . tachycardia . . . operating room . . . more steroids first . . ."

Joe lay on the bed, bathed in the light and pain.

He didn't know what time it was. He tried to focus his eyes, and they wouldn't focus, and his arms hurt, and his throat hurt, and he gagged, and his throat hurt more, and his head hurt, and he sat on the rock in the foggy valley.

Joe!

Joe!

The resident's voice poked at him, caught him, pulled.

Joe!

Joe!

Joe resisted the world of pain, but the resident's voice was a wind that blew away the fog, made Anmar vanish, created lapping waves on the sea of pain. Joe fought, hating the resident, fearing the pain.

Joe!

Joe, look at the ceiling.

Joe, squeeze my fingers.

Joe, what's two times two?

Four, leave me alone, four, four, four, go away, go away, go away, go away . . .

Time had no features, except for the punctuating visits by the resident. A woman in a white uniform hovered somewhere nearby, and sometimes she touched him.

Sometimes she hurt him by moving him, or inserting needles under his skin, but he understood that she needed to do those things. She didn't do it for pleasure, like the resident did.

Each time the resident came, Joe fought, but the resident had gone to school for years to learn every painful point on the human body. He could pull him from the valley with a simple, excruciating touch. And he never, ever, left Joe alone.

There was a clock, but Joe couldn't make his eyes focus on its face. He was afraid to ask the nurse or the resident for the time. Somehow, they would use it to hurt him. Absently, at first, but then with growing resentment, he wondered how much time had passed, how many quarters of school he had missed because of the sadistic doctors and their terrible experiments.

They kept talking about steroids. Joe thought that should ring a bell, but it didn't. Steroids? What were steroids?

Was that what they were using to cause the pain?

There was a noise above him, and the nurse injected something into a tube that ran into his arm. Then the fog curled around the bed, hiding the nurse and closing out the pain.

The blue rims of the mountains stuck up through the fog, and Joe sat on the rock.

On top of everything else, the school year was completely ruined. Ruined! Why couldn't they see how important it was for Joe to get back to school?

Joe!

Joe!

Stubbornly, without hope, he fought. The sadistic fingers reached into the inner part of his thigh, and brought him back.

Sometimes there was just one resident, and sometimes there was a whole bunch of them, except some were older. The way it worked, as nearly as Joe could figure out, was that the older guys planned the tortures and told the young ones how to keep Joe from dying in the process.

They didn't want him to die, he knew that. They can't experiment on you any more if you die.

If Joe were smart, perhaps he would resist them even in that. Death might be sweet, it might be like the foggy valley, far from the pain, except Joe didn't want to die. Despite everything. Despite the pain, he didn't want to die.

Always, the voices talked about steroids.

Why? What were steroids?

If only there were someone to talk to. He might be able to get a message out. But there was no one.

Most of what he knew about his situation he gleaned by eavesdropping. Unfortunately, his medical background was weak. He knew a lot about biology and botany, but that didn't equip him to understand a word like "atelectasis."

He didn't have a medical background but he was smart, and he listened carefully, and paid attention to context. Finally, he realized what it meant. Atelectasis. He had a collapsed lung.

". . . and give him some more steroids . . ."

He still couldn't figure out what "steroids" were. But from the context in which the doctors used the word, he was able to dope out that they were somehow central to what was going on.

Sometimes a whole lot of doctors crowded into the room and one of the older ones called him back from the cold, foggy valley and made him look up at the ceiling. Then the doctor would direct burning shafts of light into his eyes.

Mother!

Mother, take me out of here!

There were several residents, but the evil one had fingers that were long and sharp, and there was an especially hard edge in his voice. His breath smelled foul. When he pinched, he pinched hard, harder than he needed to, reaching into the valley and snatching Joe back to the world of light and pain.

Joe couldn't protect himself.

He was no better than a slave. He might as well be chained down.

He sat on the rock in the fog and thought about it.

What kind of a person became a brain surgeon?

He hadn't thought of that before. Why hadn't he thought of that?

While he was in the valley, they stuck something in his mouth, down his windpipe, and when their voices blew away the fog, their conversations told him he was on a respirator.

He had lost still another option. Now he couldn't even scream.

Joe?

Joe!

Look at me, Joe.

Look up, Joe.

The light probed into his eyes, and it hurt, it hurt, it hurt.

Edema meant swelling. His brain was swelling. The doctors were telling each other that his brain was swelling.

In the foggy valley, Joe considered the information. Was it important? He didn't know.

". . . and more steroids."

It hurt. Time passed. Joe had no sense of how much time.

When no one was watching, he practiced opening just one eye. If he did that, and if he thought very hard about what he was doing, he could see the clock on the wall. The only thing was, he didn't know if it was night or day.

The room was white, bright, ceramic, metallic, hard. Fluorescent lights reflected from stainless-steel surfaces and glinted from dial faces. The dials jerked rhythmically, biologically, but the numbers they recorded were from the cold world of mathematics and physics.

There were no dials for the pain.

Joe! Open your eyes, Joe.

Sometimes Joe's parents stood by the bed and Joe tried to tell them about the sadistic resident, but they didn't seem to understand. They shushed him like a baby and told him not to try to talk, that just meant he was getting better.

Dr. Murray said so, Joe. You're getting better.

Joe sat on the rock and concluded that the doctors had somehow gotten to his parents, put pressure on them, brainwashed them.

Joe floated into the valley and the resident pulled him back again. He wallowed in the pain and listened to the voices.

What was a "pulmonary infiltrate"?

A lot of the words sounded like they described bacteria. One of the voices, an older one, kept saying, *I want you to give him every antibiotic you've ever heard of.*

Joe was sick.

They had cut a hole in his head and carved something out. They had stuck needles in his brain. And now they were worried. Their experiments had gone too far, and they were frightened.

Joe was sick, perhaps beyond hope, and that made him sad. He wanted to live, despite everything. He hoped they felt guilty, and he desperately wished that he could hurt them back.

Again and again, the demonic resident took him downstairs to the CAT-scanner.

And everything hurt.

It hurt so bad that he wanted to pull the tube out of his nose, and the thing out of his throat, and scream. But he was too weak, and somehow he knew it wouldn't help.

". . . more steroids. And I'll write an order for Dilantin and phenobarbital."

Joe's mouth was dry, and the stomach tube gagged him.

It was never dark.

Sometimes he longed for the dark.

The fog swirled, like the fog around Mordor, far from the land of the Hobbits, where Frodo and his faithful Samwise struggled with the evil Sauron. And somewhere in the distance was Gandalf. Or was it Anmar?

Anmar.

Joe!

It hurt, and then the resident came and used his long, expert fingers to hurt him some more.

The resident was ugly.

Joe stared at the man's sharp face, hating it.

Joe!

We're going to the CAT-scanner, Joe.

Stop hurting me, please! The hatred burned brightly at the focus of the helplessness and the pain.

Slowly, flickering in and out, a resolve grew.

I won't take any more.

I'm going to hit him.

I'm not very strong, but he won't be expecting it.

Joe imagined himself swinging his arm, turning his body, ripping things, probably. He knew he would hurt himself more than he would hurt the resident, but he didn't care.

It'll be worth it.

With the passage of time, the vision of revenge filled his mind and absorbed his energy. He lay in the pain, oblivious to it for the first time, wrapped in the anticipation.

I don't care what they do to me. The next time he puts his face down here, I'm going to hit him.

Slowly, he began to drift back toward the foggy valley. But this time, he stopped himself.

No!

He must not drift away. If he drifted away, he wouldn't be alert enough to hit the resident.

Joe forced himself to concentrate, to stay in the world of pain, but the time passed slowly. He watched the minute hand of the big wall clock, counted the clicks and listened to the burbles of the suction device.

Somewhere, in another cell, someone coughed painfully.

Look at the ceiling, think about the pain, don't think about Anmar. Forget about the cool, soothing fog of the valley. Think how shocked the resident will be when your fist slams into his ugly, ugly face.

Joe might be weak, but he had the element of surprise and he had his hatred. The hatred glowed warm, like the fires in the cracks of doom, and Anmar was there.

Anmar.

The fog curled across the floor of the valley, and all his friends from all the books and dreams and games were there, safe in the fog, far from pain.

As he slept, the nurse monitored the dials and replaced the almost empty bag of glucose solution over the bed. Outside, dawn turned the clouds from black to gray. The resident came in and leaned on the counter, discussing Joe with the nurse.

Definitely, more steroids.

The resident's face was tired and haggard from the sleepless night. But before he left, he stopped by the boy's bed and stood quietly for a moment.

Perhaps he should check the neurological signs again. But Joe looked so content.

No.

He would skip it, for the moment. The kid was improving.

Let him sleep.

CHAPTER
EIGHTEEN

WHEN DR. DUCKER WAS ON CALL, HE SLEPT WITH AN EAR FOR THE telephone. It rang at 2:25 A.M.

His hand automatically shot out from under the covers and lifted the receiver in the middle of the first ring, but he was almost too late. On the other side of the bed, Barbara stirred and rolled over. He squinted at the clock.

"Ducker," he whispered into the telephone.

The chief neurosurgeon listened to the senior resident's report. A man in his early thirties apparently had an intracranial hemorrhage in a convenience store, had been rushed to a nearby hospital, and had been transferred to the University of Maryland. The fellow was barely conscious now, but his heartbeat, breathing, blood pressure and other vital signs were stable. He had no history of heart or artery disease.

The odds were, it was one of three things: a burst aneurysm, a stroke, or an arteriovenous malformation. If it were either of the first two, the blood pressure would probably have been high. So most likely it was an AVM.

Richard was the right age for an AVM to start causing trouble, and the symptoms were right. Dr. Ducker instructed the resident to monitor the patient carefully, and to call back if he got any worse.

The neurosurgeon hung up the telephone carefully, making no unnecessary noise. Then he lay for a moment in the darkness.

If it was an AVM, it was better to wait. When you opened a head right after an AVM bleed, the torn vessel might open up again. Even if it didn't, the brain tissue would be inflamed and angry, and there would be blood all over the place. There was always a risk in a case like that, always a risk of touching something you shouldn't.

Given the option, Dr. Ducker would wait a week, or even ten days. But if the patient got worse, he wouldn't have the option.

An AVM was a monster, even under the best of circumstances. It began before birth, with a tiny opening between a vein and an artery, but it didn't cause a problem then. The infant's veins were in perfect shape. They could withstand the unusually high pressure.

But by the time the patient had gotten to the age of this fellow, the vein had stretched and swelled. Auxiliary veins had developed to relieve some of the pressure, and now they, too, had enlarged. Eventually the tangled network of veins had turned into a thin-walled balloon with octopus tentacles that stretched off in all directions. The wall of the balloon had grown thinner and thinner and thinner, until now it had developed a leak.

An AVM, by the time it bled, was very fragile and fiendishly dangerous. One of Dr. Ducker's AVM patients had called her malformation a monster. Dr. Ducker agreed.

In theory, at least, removing an AVM was a straightforward neurosurgical project. You located the area where the monster was being fed by the artery and you used a clip to shut off the flow. That deflated the monster, and then it could be teased free of the brain.

But you had to know exactly where you were, and where the monster was, or you'd miss one of the feeders and Big Red would come after you. Then it was a race to see if you could find the hidden bleeder and clamp it before the patient died.

The resident had said the patient's name was, what . . . Richard. If Richard had an AVM, Dr. Ducker would probably have to go in and get it before it bled again. But not tonight, not if he could help it.

He'd get it later, when the brain itself wasn't already angry. Later, after he had taken every possible kind of X-ray, when he knew exactly where the monster was and where its tentacles led, and had figured out exactly how to approach it.

That decided, Tom Ducker went instantly back to sleep. When his alarm went off about three hours later, he awoke with Richard still at the front of his mind.

The resident was standing at the nurses' station when he saw Dr. Ducker get off the elevator shortly before seven-thirty that morning. He immediately joined his chief and walked with him toward the Neurosurgical Division office.

Richard was no worse, he told Dr. Ducker. But he was no better, either. Stable. The resident said the patient already had been to the CAT-scanner. The films were on Dr. Ducker's desk.

In his office, Dr. Ducker removed the negatives from the brown envelope and held each one up to the window.

It was definitely an intracranial bleed. He could see the huge dark shadow in the left hemisphere, about midway down in the temporal lobe. No wonder Richard was partly paralyzed. To judge from the size of the blood clot, it was a wonder that he was stable.

There was no sign of the monster, though. The hospital's CAT-scanner, for all its remarkable attributes, was nearly useless when it came to revealing the location of blood vessels. To do that, the X-ray people would have to insert a dye into Richard's vessels, then snap their pictures while the stuff filled the arteries and squirted into the monster.

An angiogram, as it was called, would outline the AVM and its tentacles clearly. But Dr. Ducker didn't want to order an angiogram yet. Not until the brain had had a few days to heal. But watch him closely, Dr. Ducker told the resident.

"If he starts to go downhill, we'll have to operate in a hurry."

"Yes sir," the resident said. Also, he added, Dr. Ducker needed to talk to the patient's wife. She was pretty distraught. Also, she was expecting a baby. Any day now.

"A baby?"

"Yes sir, a baby."

Dr. Ducker picked up one of the CAT-scan films, and held it back up to the window. The clot was huge.

CHAPTER
NINETEEN

JEAN MET TONY MASTROSTEPHANO AT A VFW DANCE. SHE HAD BEEN very pretty that night, certainly Tony thought so, and then thirty years passed. There had been two children. And in the end she sat with him, and hurt for him, when the neurologist said he would soon die.

But Jean didn't delude herself.

For one thing, the doctors and nurses were honest and forthright with her. They told her it would be easier to face it squarely. Or perhaps she told them that, by the way she held her body and asked her questions.

Anyway, they told her everything. To have glioblastoma multiforme was to die, quickly. Always. Without exception.

Glioblastoma multiforme. What a terrible name.

There were pamphlets for those close to people like Tony, who were going to die. The federal government put them out, and so did the Association for Brain Tumor Research. Jean read everything she could find.

They were all written down to perhaps a junior high school level, and there were a lot of euphemisms, but Jean got the intended message.

Even noncancerous tumors in the brain often killed, because the surgeons couldn't get all of them and they grew back. Cancers were even worse; they couldn't be stopped no matter how much was removed.

No therapy worked well on brain cancer, but some tumors grew back faster than others. Glioblastoma multiforme grew back quicker than the rest. Jean read, and she understood that Tony was going to die.

But she also understood Tony.

She had seen his face when the neurologist had told him the news.

She sensed his mind accepting the words, extracting their individual meanings, reaching the obvious conclusion . . . and then summarily rejecting it.

The doctor said it, but Tony didn't hear it.

In the beginning, the neurologist had been in a big hurry to get the operation done, but when the neurosurgeon looked at the scans, his instinct was different. He wanted to wait.

Tumors were usually taken out with a little suction device, he explained. But the best way to operate on the brain was not to touch it, and the hospital would soon have a new surgical tool that would allow him, almost, to do that. It was a laser, and it would burn away the tumor with a beam of light.

The laser would be set up in just a few days, and by waiting . . . who knows? With the laser, he might be able to get more of the tumor.

Tony was more than willing to agree to the delay. He understood he needed to have an operation, but that didn't mean he had to want it. It was like a dentist's appointment, only worse. There was a part of his mind that made it want to go away, for the appointment to be cancelled, for World War III to begin. He didn't even want to think about it. Jean didn't blame him.

Jean knew, intellectually, that a time would come when her husband would have to face it. She could make him understand, if she had to. She could sit him down and say *Tony, you have to listen* and he would listen. She would tell him he would die, and then, she was confident, he would hear.

She knew she might have to do that.

But not now, not right before Thanksgiving.

So, after ten days in the hospital, Tony came home without his operation.

High doses of steroids had reduced the swelling inside his brain, so that it no longer pressed on the nerves. With the pressure gone, there were no more headaches. But he wasn't his old self.

Jean resolved not to take off work any more than necessary (she would need the time later on), so she was away most weekdays.

While she was gone he watched television. At no time did he complain about not being allowed to go back to work, and that was unlike him.

The family was together on Thanksgiving, but the joy was self-conscious and forced. A few days later Bryn Mawr Hospital called. The neurosurgeon's laser was in operation, and Tony was on the schedule for the morning of December 8.

The day after the call, Jean took Tony to the hospital. Two days later, she sat in the waiting room while they operated on his brain.

She waited a long time, and the ashtray next to where she was sitting slowly filled with cigarette butts. Finally the neurosurgeon came in and sat down beside her.

It was exactly what they thought it was.

The neurosurgeon said they had removed as much of it as they could, and in that sense the operation was a success. Now it would have to be followed by X-ray therapy.

Gently but firmly, he made certain Jean understood that the prognosis was unchanged. The operation might keep Tony alive a little longer, perhaps a year. Perhaps a year and a half. Longer than that was unlikely.

Please don't tell him, Jean pleaded. It was her choice, the doctor said. *I'll tell him.* Later. When there is no other choice. Or when he wants to know.

But at work she was honest with her co-workers—honestly desperate.

Jean worked as a secretary in the counseling department at the high school where her son was a student, and the story of her tragic situation was passed from person to person. There was an upwelling of sympathy and support. One of Jean's closest friends worked in the library, and she had a sister who was in nursing school down at the University of Maryland, in Baltimore. She promised to ask her sister for information and advice.

Jean didn't keep the secret from her children, either. Mother, son and daughter supported one another, and together they supported Tony as he recovered at home. No matter what, they promised themselves grimly, it would be a good Christmas.

For Jean, the secret was a terrible burden—just having it, not sharing that part of things with Tony. She wasn't in the habit of keeping secrets from her husband, and she felt guilty every time she lied to him.

It was not that the lying was a difficult thing to accomplish. It wasn't. After the operation, he had been quick to accept her words at face value, quick to believe that it hadn't been glioblastoma multiforme after all.

The doctors had made a mistake. It hadn't been cancer. It had been something else, something benign, and the surgeons had gotten it all. Now all that had to be done was take some medicine and get a few X-ray treatments.

It was depressingly easy.

From that moment on, Jean lived in constant fear that Tony would discover her lie. Yet she dreaded even more that he *wouldn't* find out, and that she would have to tell him . . .

But not today. Please, not today.

She took great precautions. When she wrote away for information on glioblastoma multiforme, she asked that it be sent to her at the school. She instructed the doctors and nurses to call her at work; never at home.

Occasionally, co-workers passed along newspaper clippings about glioblastoma multiforme. But not often. In the first place, there weren't very many such articles. In the second place, they weren't the kind of thing you show to a woman who is about to become a widow, not unless you were her very close friend. The clippings were all very depressing.

At home, Tony sat and watched television, and the days passed. Sometimes one of his co-workers came by to take him to the X-ray therapy sessions. In the evenings, friends visited.

After the radiation treatments, chunks of his hair fell out. The headaches came back, and the doctors gave him more steroids. Christmas was doggedly joyful.

When she returned to her job after the Christmas vacation, Jean found a message to contact her friend in the school library. She picked up the telephone and returned the call. The librarian said she had talked to her sister at nursing school, and her sister had sent her a publication containing a story about glioblastoma.

The publication was *Happenings*, the campus newspaper at the University of Maryland's medical school complex in Baltimore. It featured an article about a Dr. Michael Salcman, a neurosurgeon at the medical school.

Cancer, Dr. Salcman said in the story, was particularly sensitive to heat. Jean read that Dr. Salcman had inserted a little heating device into the head of a brain tumor patient. He thought it might help in treating glioblastoma multiforme, a deadly brain cancer.

Yes, he said, the procedure was highly experimental, but it could be justified in cases of a uniformly fatal disease like glioblastoma multiforme.

Jean read the article again, looking for hope.

Clearly, there wasn't very much hope. But if there was even some . . .

It was the hopelessness of glioblastoma multiforme that made it necessary to lie. But if there was any hope at all, it would give him strength. The smallest, most fragile thread of hope would eliminate the need to lie.

She read the article once more, and then again. Finally, she picked up the telephone. For the first time since that terrible hour in the neurologist's office, Jean was doing something positive. Instantly, she felt better.

The information operator gave her the telephone number of the University of Maryland Hospital. Eventually she reached Sharon Wellslager, Dr. Salcman's secretary.

Jean didn't get much encouragement from Sharon. Sharon told her, nicely but firmly, that Tony's chances of becoming a patient of Dr. Salcman's were somewhat remote. No, not impossible, just remote.

Dr. Salcman, Sharon said, was picking his cases very carefully. The standard treatment for glioblastoma multiforme was to operate once, and that meant that Dr. Salcman couldn't offer microwave treatment until the patient had had the operation and the tumor had returned. He wouldn't implant a microwave antenna unless it was a last resort, a desperate, final gamble.

Put bluntly, Dr. Salcman wouldn't even consider treating Tony until Tony's own doctor had written him off.

He had, Jean assured her.

There was something else, then.

She explained that doctors disagreed on the classification of glioblastoma multiforme. Dr. Salcman only used the microwave on those he agreed had glioblastoma multiforme, the really bad ones, so that the results of the study couldn't be challenged. So he would have to see Tony's medical records.

Also, the tumor would have to be in the right place. Dr. Salcman didn't have very much experience in warming the heat-sensitive brain cells, and there were places he simply refused to place the antenna. If Tony's cancer had grown into one of those places, forget it.

Finally, another "if."

The microwave project was an experimental one, and the first instrument had been put together for one or two operations, enough to prove it could be done without harming the patient. Now Dr. Samaras, the project's engineer, had had it all torn apart. He was building another model, a better one, with a lot of safety features.

The new model was supposed to be better, but it wasn't working yet. Sharon was vague about what the problem was and Jean wouldn't have understood it if it had been explained.

So Sharon hadn't encouraged her, but neither had she said Dr. Salcman wouldn't see Tony. Sharon had tried to make the chances seem slim, very slim, but she'd had no grasp of Jean's desperation.

Jean hung up the telephone, her spirits high. Suddenly, there was much to do. On Sharon's instructions, she made arrangements to have Tony's medical records forwarded to Dr. Salcman, who would then decide whether or not Tony's was the correct kind of case for the experiment.

That meant she had to call the hospital where he had gotten the CAT scan, the hospital where the surgery had been performed, and the neurologist who had made the diagnosis.

A few days after she called the hospital to have their records forwarded to Dr. Salcman, Jean took Tony to the radiation clinic for a treatment. The nurses there were friendly and helpful, and they always took time to chat with Tony whenever he came in.

This time, Jean and Tony had only been in the clinic for a few minutes when one of the nurses saw Tony and came over.

Oh, Mr. Mastrostephano! Hello! We just sent your pathology slides down to the University of Maryland.

Tony looked at her, blankly. Slides? University of Maryland?

Jean stood behind him, furiously shaking her head and screaming, silently, with her lips, no, no, no, no!

For an instant, the nurse appeared confused. Then she understood. She hesitated, then looked down at her clipboard.

Oh. I've made an error. It must have been someone else I was thinking of, yes, right here, it was someone else. Well. How are you today?

I'm just fine, Tony said. Great.

Jean's adrenaline level dropped slowly.

A week later, there was another incident.

Getting Tony's records to Dr. Salcman had proved to be more difficult than Jean had anticipated. The bureaucracy was terrible.

One problem was that the radiology department at the hospital wouldn't release his CAT scans without the permission of the neurologist who first made the diagnosis. Jean called the neurologist from the school.

The doctor agreed to straighten things out and get the records released. He would call back, he promised, as soon as it was taken care of.

As soon as he got the chance, the neurologist called the hospital and told the radiology department to release the records. Then he looked for Jean's number.

He couldn't find the slip of paper he'd written it on, but he had

Tony's chart in front of him. There were two numbers there. He dialed the first one.

At home, Tony picked up the telephone.

I just wanted to let you know, he told Tony. I signed the release for your CAT scans today. You can pick them up at the hospital anytime.

Release? Tony hesitated.

Oh. Well, he said. Thanks.

That night, puzzled, he told Jean about the telephone call.

Jean was peeling potatoes. As Tony talked, the peeler slipped and cut into the tip of her index finger. Quickly, she put the bleeding hand in her apron pocket.

She forced herself to be calm, to sound nonchalant.

I can't imagine . . . who knows? I'll have to call and find out if we were supposed to pick them up for some reason, she said, sounding uninterested. Maybe he had the wrong patient.

Maybe.

Something like that.

Tony guessed so.

The conversation lapsed, and the subject changed.

The next day Jean went to the hospital, picked up the records, and sent them off to Dr. Salcman. Then there was nothing left to do but wait for Sharon to call. Days passed.

Why was it taking Dr. Salcman so long?

Jean tried to make herself be patient, but in a few days she called Baltimore from work. It took time, Sharon counseled her. Be patient.

A few days later, Jean called again.

It took them forever to get and assemble all the records they needed, and then it took them forever to look at them. Cancer rounds were on Wednesday, Sharon said. The doctors were planning to review Tony's records this coming Wednesday.

But they didn't, and that meant it would be next Wednesday for certain. But next Wednesday came and went, and there was no telephone call.

There was no hurry, Sharon said. The machine still wasn't working right, anyway. She said she didn't know what the problem was. All she knew was that Dr. Samaras and Dr. Salcman were beginning to act very frustrated about it.

She tried to reassure Mrs. Mastrostephano. It wouldn't be long. Next Wednesday.

January became February, February became March.

Finally, as April approached, the call came. Jean stopped typing and picked up the telephone.

Sharon was on the line. When Jean recognized the voice, her heart began pounding.

Sharon said a lot of things, but the thing Jean heard was *yes*. Well, a qualified yes. Dr. Salcman would examine Tony. Then, maybe. If the tumor was still in a good place. If the machine worked. Jean hung up the telephone, numb. Sharon had said "if," and "if" meant there was hope.

A co-worker who had overheard the conversation got up, came over, and threw her arms around Jean. Soon, there were several people there, congratulating her.

Jean's mind worked furiously. Her son needed to know, and her daughter.

And finally, Tony.

Jean sat back down in front of the typewriter and scrolled in a clean piece of paper. Her foot neared the dictaphone's switch, then hesitated.

What would she say to Tony?

She picked up the telephone and dialed her daughter's telephone number. It would help, Jean explained, if she could have some company when she told him.

At the other end of the telephone there was a moment of silence.

Mother, please, don't make me be there.

Afterward, then?

The evening had been planned, weeks before. Company was coming that night. Jean had made the arrangements and looked forward to conversations with old friends, but now everything was changed.

Her daughter and daughter's husband arrived early, and that helped. When the chimes rang, Jean opened the door with a smile.

Somehow, she kept the smiling mask in place, and the evening passed. Finally, she and Tony showed their guests to the door. Then Jean, Tony, their daughter and her husband sat alone in the Mastro-stephano living room.

Jean suggested that she and Tony go to the den, but he demurred. He was full from dinner, comfortable, content.

Come on, Tony, there's something I want to tell you.

His daughter and son-in-law sat silently, uncomfortably.

Why can't you tell me here?

She held her ground.

I want to tell you privately.

Tony frowned at her.

You're going to give me bad news?

No, no, I just want to talk to you. Please?

Tony got up and followed her to the den. They sat together on the couch.

Tony, I've never held anything back from you. You know that. So I don't know how you're going to take this, but I've been lying, telling little white lies.

They didn't get all the tumor. Not with the operation, not with the drugs, not with the radiation. It's a very bad cancer, and it's already coming back.

Tony's face was blank.

I thought I was getting better.

The words were slow, puzzled, and they hurt Jean terribly. She sat very still for a moment, and then she spoke again.

Tony, there's a doctor in Baltimore.

Tony looked at her.

There's a doctor in Baltimore who has a brand-new operation that he's doing for your kind of cancer, and he's agreed to operate on you.

He looked at her. It had been almost thirty years since he'd met her, right after the war. It was in Pennsylvania, in coal country. Things were bad then, but she had been beautiful. She was still beautiful. She had concealed it until she had something good to say.

My God, Jean, how did you do all of this?

There was absolutely no anger in his voice, just wonder, and Jean's pain abated a little. She had finally told him the truth, and the burden lifted. She watched Tony as his mind fastened on the hope she had given him.

I'm going to whip this thing, he said. *I'm going to beat it.*

TWENTY

THERE IS A TRADITION IN GEORGE SAMARAS' WORLD THAT A GOOD engineer can do almost anything with a few spare parts and a soldering iron. In that sense, Dr. Samaras was pleased with the first microwave system. It looked like a rack of hand-me-down equipment, and in fact it was—but the bioengineer had the utmost confidence in its ability to do what it was supposed to.

Or, to be more precise, he had confidence in his own ability to step in and save the situation if it didn't. He had planned it, built it, and now, inevitably, it had to be he that operated it.

The day before Dr. Salcman was to implant the antenna Dr. Samaras had to see that the equipment got transported safely from the laboratory building over to the hospital's operating suites, a half block away.

During each move he walked alongside the dolly, steadying the tall rack of equipment as it lurched down the hallway to the elevator and then along a sidewalk to the hospital. In the hospital elevator, bored patients gawked at it.

When the equipment was safely parked in a storage room across the hall from Operating Room Eleven, Dr. Samaras plugged it in and ran through a series of tests to make certain it hadn't been damaged in transit.

During the operations themselves, Dr. Samaras was almost as indispensable as the surgeon. After Dr. Salcman debulked the tumor and positioned the antenna, the bioengineer sat by the generating equipment, flipping switches and turning dials, his eyes fixed on the critical temperature monitors.

It wasn't a responsibility that Dr. Samaras could trust to anyone else. Only he knew the machine's quirks well enough to react knowledgeably in an emergency. An emergency, of course, was defined as the temperature probe getting too hot or too cool.

No such emergency occurred, of course, nor would it—as long as George Samaras was in the OR.

Each of the first patients received three doses of microwave heat. The initial treatment was given right in the operating room, and was largely a calibration run. It lasted about fifteen minutes. The next two were performed in the neurosurgical intensive care unit. They lasted an hour each.

During that hour Dr. Samaras sat, immobile and tense, his eyes on the temperature readout. The equipment hummed, almost inaudibly. Whenever the numbers changed slightly, his fingers adjusted the controls. A little more power. A little less. A little more.

By paying very close attention, Dr. Samaras could keep the temperature stable to within half a degree centigrade. That seemed crude to him, as an engineer, but the doctors thought it was pretty good.

After the first operation, Dr. Salcman was pleased. And so was Dr. Samaras. It had worked, and the patient had seemed to tolerate the heating without any side effects. The results of the second operation were similar, and again, Dr. Salcman was pleased.

Dr. Samaras was less so.

The equipment was a prototype, he explained. It wasn't built to be hauled down the sidewalk on a dolly, and sooner or later something would go wrong. When it did, Dr. Samaras would be there to catch it and avert disaster, but . . . put bluntly, the bioengineer had better things to do with his life.

The prototype had served its purpose, Dr. Samaras said. With it they had proved that they could heat a human brain without doing any detectable damage. It was time to retire it, and build something more portable. And safer. Safe enough for a technician to operate.

But there was a long backlog of dying glioblastoma multiforme patients, and Dr. Samaras let himself be talked into one more operation. Then he called a halt. No more. Not without a more trustworthy machine.

The new machine, as Dr. Samaras envisioned it, would hold the temperature perfectly steady, and would check and cross-check its own functions and shut itself down if anything went wrong. That would make it safer for the patients and, at the same time, free George Samaras.

Michael Salcman, having no choice, agreed to wait for the new machine.

When Jean Mastrostephano called, Sharon told her what she was telling all the patients and their families. She was sorry, but the microwave implants weren't being done, at the moment. The microwave machine was being worked on, rebuilt, something like that. It would be ready soon.

What was wrong with the old one? Jean asked.

Sharon didn't really know, but something was—either that, or they just wanted to make it better. Scientists did that, sometimes.

George Samaras breathed a sigh of relief. He would much rather be working in the lab than in the operating room. He didn't worry about his ability to build the machine he envisioned. After all, why should he? He was a bioengineer, and it was a classic bioengineering problem.

Step one was to think the problem through clearly, using as many brains as possible. He summoned his engineering group to the conference room adjacent to his office and laid out the situation. Hands dipped into lab-coat pockets and withdrew calculators. Symbols appeared on lined note pads. Somebody went for coffee.

Obviously, if the microwave generator had to operate perfectly, the first thing to do was identify everything that possibly could go wrong. It was all very well for a neurosurgeon to talk about how something might happen, but "something" was a poor engineering concept. The engineers wouldn't rest easy until the individual problems could be reduced to equations, numbers and computer routines.

Day after day, Dr. Samaras and his engineers convened in the conference room for brainstorming sessions designed to dredge up every possible accident, no matter how unlikely. They thought about blown fuses, and malfunctioning condensers. They thought about dumb and obvious mistakes that the machine could make, and about sophisticated and arcane ones, about part failures and software problems.

The work was creative, technical and exhausting. As the brainstorming sessions went on day after day, the laboratory's coffee consumption went up. The list of possible somethings that could go wrong grew.

They would take nothing for granted, trust nothing but the most fundamental truths of the engineer's universe. Electrons would flow through copper wire, E would equal mc squared, Ohm's law would hold firm and the power in the receptacle would be grounded, sixty-cycle, alternating current.

The longer the list of somethings grew, the more George Samaras became convinced that he had done the correct thing in refusing to do a fourth operation. The list of potential disasters was even longer than he'd guessed it would be. There were hundreds of things that could go wrong, and they could go wrong in hundreds of thousands of combinations. Each problem, once defined, had a solution designed for it, and a backup solution for that.

Finally, Dr. Samaras was convinced that his group had thought of every possible problem, and had designed machinery and computer programs to correct for them. It looked as though the new micro-wave-therapy device would be perfect.

It was taking longer than he'd anticipated, but when Dr. Salcman became impatient, Dr. Samaras soothed him. This sort of thing can get very complicated, you know. Quality science takes time.

Soon, he told Dr. Salcman.

Dr. Salcman repeated the promise to Sharon, and Sharon repeated it to Jean Mastrostephano. Soon, she told Tony. Soon.

Back in the laboratory, assembling the hardware for the microwave transmitter was a relatively minor concern. Everything the scientific team needed, except for the antenna itself, could be purchased from a scientific supply house. Hooking all the pieces together was routine . . . but you had to expect some glitches. In the laboratory, you could think about a glitch, figure it out and fix it. These would all have to be figured out and fixed, completely fixed, before the equipment was ever used on a patient.

Dr. Samaras' strategy was based on a system of not one, but four computers. One ran and monitored the generator itself, the second checked the temperature constantly and made adjustments, and the third made certain it and the other two computers were talking to one another properly.

Unless all three computers were functioning and communicating, the machine would refuse to operate.

The heart of the device was a fourth computer, the one that did the worrying. It was a fail-safe, error-checking computer, with cybernetic tentacles extending throughout the entire microwave-therapy machine.

It checked everything compulsively, a thousand times a second, and if anything was awry it instantly corrected the problem, or shut everything down. The fail-safe, error-checking computer even checked itself by doing everything twice and comparing the two results.

Finally, the fail-safe, error-checking computer did its own trouble-shooting. When something went wrong, it would examine itself and flash a message that would tell the operator what was wrong, and how to fix it.

In six months, it was finished. Dr. Salcman breathed a sigh of relief.

Dr. Samaras plugged it in. Nothing happened. Frowning, the bioengineer touched the keyboard.

The computer consulted itself for a moment, and then the answer to a Great Question appeared on the screen. The universe, the fail-safe, error-checking computer said in perfect computerese, was an imperfect place. There was, for openers, the matter of the incorrect opcode in program location F3.

The error-checking computer had found one problem, that was all. Under the circumstances, it was only natural that the fail-safe, error-checking computer would refuse to allow itself to be turned on. Dr. Samaras went right to work on it.

Sharon told Jean that she was sorry, but no, the machine wasn't ready yet. There was some kind of a problem. No, Sharon was sure it wasn't very serious, and she would call as soon as she knew anything, but she was sure it would be soon . . .

The fail-safe, error-checking computer told them what was wrong, of course. They fixed it, and told the fail-safe, error-checking computer to start itself up. But no, a few steps further away there was a misplaced binary bit in the E register.

Yup. Sure enough. There was a misplaced binary bit in the E register. The thing was never wrong. It was perfect.

Now? they asked the fail-safe, error-checking computer.

No, it replied. Not with a circular subroutine call at location 11D.

Oh.

From a computer's point of view, a perfect world can have no circular subroutines. Dr. Samaras and the technicians did what the machine told them to, and tried again. And again. And again. Weeks passed. Soon, said Dr. Samaras, soon.

Each time the scientists did what the machine told them to do, the process moved on. Each solution unmasked a new problem. Dr. Salcman collected letters from dying glioblastoma multiforme patients, and he turned them down. Sorry, he said. Soon.

Solution followed problem, problem followed solution.

Was there such a thing as perfect?

Was there always something wrong?

Finally, in a flash of inspiration, it came to him. Dr. Samaras could disconnect the disconnect device on the fail-safe, error-checking computer, so that it couldn't stop the machine from functioning. The fail-safe, error-checking computer would then produce an error message at every glitch, but it wouldn't stop the machine. That way, he could find out how many error messages there were.

He did it, and the fail-safe, error-checking computer took a long, long, time to assemble a list of errors and imperfections. The list was dismayingly long.

On the other hand, the bioengineer told himself, the complaints all consisted of the picayunish sort of i-dotting and t-crossing that one would expect of a cybernetic pedant, and they could all be readily fixed.

Finally, a year after Dr. Samaras started work on the device, Jean Mastrostephano received a call from Dr. Salcman's secretary.

Jean knew instantly that the call was important. She usually called Sharon, not vice versa.

Yes, Jean said into the telephone.

Yes, of course.

She and Tony could be there anytime. Next week would be fine. Wonderful.

Perfect.

CHAPTER
TWENTY-ONE

FOR WEEKS AFTER THE OPERATION, PAIN DOMINATED JOE TROTT'S MIND, stretching out the minutes. Life was pain interrupted by sleep, pain driven on by the sadistic resident, pain underlaid by indignity.

The pain was *right now,* and in all its urgency it masked the terror.

Joe's mind worked better, now—a little slowly, it seemed sometimes, but he had plenty of time, and he listened carefully with his one good ear, and he puzzled out what was going on. Something had happened about the operation. Something hadn't gone right.

The doctors were coming around so often because they were afraid he was going to die. Joe figured this out, and sorted through his mind for the fear that should be there. He couldn't find it. Whatever part of his brain was responsible for being afraid was too sick to be working.

All he cared about was the pain.

The minutes passed slowly in the bright room, and one nurse followed another on endless shifts. Bottle after bottle of intravenous fluid emptied into his arm. The bandages on his head grew soggy with fluid, and were changed.

He could see the clock, when he was conscious, but it didn't help orient him. Was it morning, or evening?

By the time the pain subsided, there was no longer any reason to fear imminent death. For some reason that the doctors didn't understand, he hadn't died. Now the crisis was over.

For the moment. When he was well enough to understand, they told him the news. The surgeons hadn't been able to get it all. They would have to go back in again.

By now, of course, Joe was used to surviving minute by minute and the news wasn't particularly disturbing. The second operation seemed like a long way in the future and it was enough, for the moment, not to hurt so badly.

He'd gotten pneumonia, they said.

They said the nerve leading to one side of his throat had been paralyzed, and that weakened the valve that sealed off the trachea during swallowing. The valve didn't close properly, and some of Joe's first sip of water worked its way into his lungs, where it triggered an infection . . .

That's why he was on a respirator. It kept him from drowning in phlegm.

Slowly, he improved.

After he got home, Joe calculated that he had spent ninety-nine days at the hospital, thirty-one of them in the SICU, as miserable as he had ever been in his life. Not that his recuperation at home was easy. The blinding pain in his head had gone, but it had now been replaced with back pain, a slow, burning ache that gradually got worse.

As the incision in his head healed itself, the back pain got worse. It didn't hurt quite enough for Dr. Murray to readmit Joe to the hospital, but it hurt too much for him to lead a normal life. He stretched out on the couch, or the floor, searching restlessly for a less painful position, watching the minutes turn into hours and the hours into days.

He had plenty of time to think.

The tumor had grown from the left acoustic nerve, so he was deaf in his left ear. He couldn't read, because the nerves controlling his eye movements were also involved, and he was cross-eyed. He couldn't have long conversations with visitors because his vocal cords wouldn't produce anything but a hoarse whisper. His only unimpaired sense was the hearing in his right ear.

In the hospital, the radio had been almost his only link with the outside world. At home, it always played softly in the background, telling him all about the presidential election campaign, the Iranian hostage crisis, and Preparation H.

When his attention drifted, he fantasized.

Caves.

A stalagmite rises from the floor of a cave, and a stalactite hangs from the ceiling. You can remember which is which by the fact that something has to be stuck pretty tight to hang from the ceiling. Stalactites are tight.

That way, you never forget and make a fool out of yourself in the presence of more experienced cavers.

The temperature in a deep cave is always about sixty-five degrees.

When caving, watch where you put your feet.

". . . your station for local news. A judge in Annapolis today ruled that a group of Montgomery County taxpayers may proceed with their lawsuit against former Vice-President Spiro Agnew. The taxpayers want Agnew to pay back the money he received in kickbacks while he was governor . . ."

Girls.

Girls were great fantasy material. Girls in skirts, girls in pants, girls in whatever . . . blondes, brunettes, redheads, tall girls, short girls, girls.

But even girl fantasies become tired, and worn, so Joe thought about getting rich, about getting famous, about being heroic, about Dungeons and Dragons, about his friends, about school.

Sometimes, despite the radio, despite the fantasies, he had nothing to think about but the facts.

On the one hand, he wasn't dead. On the other, this brain tumor business was far from finished. And his folks were definitely worried. They were so worried that they made Joe nervous, and he learned to put them at ease by joking about his situation.

I got a lot on my mind, he said, when it became clear that the tumor was growing again. It made everybody grin, and relax.

I've been busy, he told relatives. *Growing hair is a lot of work.*

It was easier on everybody if Joe stayed cool.

It was, in fact, easier on everybody if you didn't hate the resident . . . no, don't think about the resident. The resident was one subject Joe almost couldn't face. In hindsight, he was mortified by the hatred he had felt for the resident.

Damn! They told him he'd be sick, but they didn't tell him the steroids would make him paranoid! They should have told him that!

Joe would have slugged the poor fellow, if he could have stayed awake long enough. He was infinitely glad, now, for his sleepiness. That would have been awful. When things got so bad that you slugged your SICU resident, you had lost your cool completely.

The tumor was growing like crazy. It was already starting to push its way out of the hole they left in the back of his skull. A soft lump extended outward, a little bit at first, then farther, until it was the size of a goose egg. And it was very soft.

The doctors were interested in the soft lump. They touched it, delicately, and ordered more CAT scans. Joe was given to understand that the lump should be treated with care.

Fact: Dr. Long said specifically that it wasn't malignant.

Question: Did acoustic tumors ever turn malignant?

Never.

Or, almost never.

Dr. Long wouldn't lie to him. He was certain of that. Positive.

Was he really? *How certain was he?*

Nothing is ever one hundred percent certain.

Nothing.

Ever.

The tumor was coming back.

Cancer comes back.

". . . a black poodle with a rhinestone collar, answering to the name Muffin, lost in the vicinity of Roland Park Country School. There is a hundred dollar reward for . . ."

Joe fantasized about caves, and outer space, and his thoughts drifted toward school, then back again.

Death was to be avoided, but it wasn't just life that Joe wanted. He wanted normalcy. If he had to risk his life for normalcy, well, then, he would risk it.

Life was less precious anyway, when your back hurt all the time.

The doctors said they didn't know why his back hurt.

Metastasis? A secondary tumor in the spine?

It was a fair question.

". . . intermittent rain and twenty-mile-an-hour winds . . ."

As a freshman, he'd bought his rat hat, and he'd intended to keep it. He had thought he might want to bronze it one day, after he became successful. Everybody had told him those would be the best days of his life, and everybody had been right.

At some indeterminate, unremembered moment he quit looking back to the last operation and started looking forward to the next one.

"When can we get this thing over with?" he demanded. "I've got to get back to school."

Later, the doctors said. Get better. We'll see you in two weeks. More physical therapy.

Noooooo . . . not quite yet.

In two more weeks, and more physical therapy.

Come back in ten days, and more physical therapy.

Finally, the doctors agreed he was ready. His parents brought him to the hospital. Joe insisted on walking in, unassisted. They'd put him in a wheelchair soon enough.

Joe was very co-operative, and very cool, and this time he knew the routine. When the nurses came around with the needles, he rolled up his sleeve and held out his arm.

"You realize, of course, that this is interfering with my hairdresser's appointment . . ."

Joe put up with it all, and fretted over the passing school term. It took them a week to get their act together, but finally they set a date. Tomorrow, they said.

Tomorrow.

It would be good to have it finished, one way or the other.

But first, there was tonight.

It was dark outside. His parents had come and gone.

Joe lay on the bed, passing the minutes, waiting to get it over with, thinking about school, not death.

Still, death was an interesting subject.

Death, strictly speaking, was the absence of biological life. Death was when the brain died, but did the mind die with it?

Fact: Joe's mind couldn't imagine not being able to imagine. If there was no place in the mind for a concept, then that concept had to be wrong.

Fact: Joe's universe was coded in his brain. When his brain ceased to exist, so did his universe.

Well.

If the universe ceased to exist, then Joe would simply have to get along without it.

Fact: Tomorrow morning, early, they're going to come and get me, put me on a cart, roll me down the hall, inject me with something that makes me goofy. They're going to cut my head open, and I'm going to wake up, if at all, in the bright SICU room.

There was every reason to be frightened. It was abnormal and irrational not to be frightened.

So why wasn't he?

He wished he could see well enough to read a book.

A nurse appeared, carrying a pill. She put it down by the water.

"Is everything okay? Can I get you anything?"

"I'm fine, but . . ."

The nurse paused by the door.

"I'm a little concerned about the steroids."

The nurse came back in. "Yes?"

"The last time, the steroids changed my personality. I didn't know that until later. Would you make sure everyone knows that if I start acting strange, it's only the steroids?"

"Don't worry about it," the nurse reassured him. "We deal with that all the time. We understand."

After she left, Joe got up and went to the bathroom to brush his teeth.

Gotta prevent cavities.

Were there cavities in Anmar's world?

Joe had never asked the question.

I ought to be scared.

I must have a hole in my head.

On the other hand, it doesn't make it any different if you blow your cool. Everything will happen just the same, anyway.

He rinsed out the toothbrush, carefully, and returned to his bed.

Why should I be afraid? After all, I'm going to sleep through the whole thing.

He lay back, closed one eye, and looked at the ceiling.

How many other people were on this floor, in this hospital, waiting, as he waited, to get it over with?

The hospital noises died down at night, but for someone who had trained himself to get most of his information through his one good ear, it was never quiet.

From down the hall, there was the clatter of stainless steel against stainless steel. Two residents paused briefly outside his door, talking in long words about some woman's back. From somewhere, far away, there was the warble of an ambulance.

Well, what the heck . . . it'll be a load off my mind.

He took the pill and turned off the light.

CHAPTER
TWENTY-TWO

OUTSIDE IT WAS DARK AND COLD. TWELVE FLOORS BELOW, TRAFFIC crawled along Baltimore streets. A helicopter circled far above, lights flashing, then settled toward the roof of a parking garage.

Tony lit a cigarette. Unconsciously, Jean reached for her own pack. She would have to slow down sometime, but not now.

Tony was talking about going back to work, about all that computer stuff. Jean monitored the sentences, but she didn't really listen. Her interest in computers was minimal, except that they were important to Tony.

Hope.

Dr. Salcman had been very honest with her all along. The microwave antenna was just being safety-tested, that was all. There was absolutely no evidence that Tony would be cured. Realistically, the young surgeon had said to her, there was no hope of a cure.

No hope, except . . . had there been hope for the first child cured of leukemia?

Dr. Salcman didn't know it *wouldn't* work, did he?

No, he didn't, and that fact was all Jean needed for her husband. It gave him something to do while he waited to die. It allowed him to talk to her now, as the operation approached, about computers.

If he couldn't talk about computers, what would he talk about? Death?

Jean's mind returned to her husband as his monologue switched from computers to lobster tails. Yes, she promised. When he gets home she'll prepare lobster tails, as many as he wants.

Better lobster tails than death.

The best reasonable expectation, Dr. Salcman had said, was for perhaps another year. The operation itself, by removing the regrown tumor, could provide that even without the microwave procedure.

But the hope was more important than the year. If Tony never woke up after the operation, it would nonetheless have been worth it. He would never have had to live a moment without hope.

At least there were no secrets between them. The lying had been difficult for Jean, though she had known she had to do it. It had conflicted with the rule that a good wife doesn't deceive her husband, and she was relieved, finally, when he knew the worst.

After that night of truth in the den, she could share her collection of newspaper clippings about the doctor in Baltimore, who didn't give up on glioblastoma multiforme patients. She could get the calls at home, and share them with Tony. She could reminisce about how worried she had been every time someone almost revealed the secret. Now she could talk with him about her calls to Sharon, and now she could share the hope she had nurtured so carefully over the months.

After the operation was scheduled, Jean called the school and arranged to take time off. It had been intelligent of her to save her vacation time. The school, as usual, was wonderful, offering no complaints about the short notice.

She also had to make arrangements to stay somewhere close to Tony. A motel in Baltimore was out of the question. The money might be needed later. So she called her sister in Delaware, a forty-five-minute drive from Baltimore, and that problem was solved.

Somebody had to take care of her son. Yes, of course, her daughter would do that. There was a dinner engagement to cancel. She would have to get her checkbook balanced, so that she could know exactly how much money she had in any emergency.

She would have to anticipate the possibility of all emergencies.

Did the car need servicing?

She would wear a skirt and blouse.

Jean had planned carefully, and nothing had gone wrong. Now, finally, there was only tonight, and tomorrow morning.

The minutes passed slowly as she half-listened to Tony talk of computers, lobster tails, swimming, football, the Philadelphia Eagles, twenty-two men out on a field, fighting over a little odd-shaped ball.

Outside, the pollution made bright halos around the sodium-vapor streetlights.

"Jean, I'm going to whip this thing."

That's what he always said. He said it to his friends, to the doctors and the nurses, even to Jean.

There was always the one in a million chance, the crazy statistic. Perhaps he might.

With hope, and love, they would get through the night, and the morning, and whatever might follow.

CHAPTER
TWENTY-THREE

RICHARD STOOD IN THE ROARING SHOWER AND LET THE HOT WATER massage his body. The steam wafted into his nostrils, and the sound of the water muffled the noises of the hospital.

Dr. Ducker had told Richard not to eat supper the night before the operation. Richard had been too nervous to eat, anyway. Besides, the food at the University of Maryland Hospital ranged from mediocre to intolerable. He was probably missing a microwaved sawdust patty and a side order of drowned spinach. That was not exactly a complaint. The food was lousy here, but the institution more than compensated with shower facilities that were far better than what he had at home.

The bathroom walls were done in shiny tile that was unmarred by stains or cracks, and the faucets provided very good control of water flow. The shower stall was also equipped with sturdy chromium bars. The second day after his bleed, when they had finally allowed him to take a shower, he had needed to cling to the bars to remain upright.

Now he was much better. He could stand up without holding on to anything. Tomorrow, he would be worse again.

Thoughtfully, Richard grasped a bar of soap, stepped out of the water flow, and scrubbed first under his left arm and then his right.

Tomorrow he could be dead.

Dr. Ducker hadn't said it exactly that way, and he didn't dwell on it, but Richard had gotten the message.

Richard's brain had worked very slowly during those first few painful days. He apparently looked stupid, because people sometimes spoke to him more clearly than usual, and they explained things very, very simply. But he hadn't been stupid at all, just slow. It had taken him a while to think it all through, but he'd had nothing else to do but think.

He remembered going to the fast-foods store, and struggling to take the 7-Up out of the cooler. He remembered the lights of the ambulance, and he remembered, and resented, the doctor in the emergency room.

The man had tried to dump him off the stretcher.

Well, maybe he hadn't tried. But Richard had been sick and frightened and paralyzed, and he'd felt himself sliding. The terror was instant and awful, and he had clawed at the stretcher with his good hand, seeking support.

The recollection made Richard angry, even now. After all the hard years, after struggling with the habit, then the poverty, then the lack of education . . . after overcoming all that, and then after falling suddenly ill, how unfair to be terrorized, to be deprived so casually of his dignity.

He took a deep breath, replaced the bar of soap, stepped back into the shower and let the stream of water wash the suds away. The anger went with it.

Absently, Richard reached down and increased the hot water flow a tiny bit. Then he turned his back to the shower head and let the thousands of hot little needles pound down onto his shoulders.

He had regained consciousness with his right side still paralyzed and his head hurting. He had been confused for a while, but then he had understood: He was in a hospital.

He had slept a lot at first, except when they had moved him onto a cart and taken him someplace, usually to stick his head into something. Once they had put his head under a huge X-ray machine, and then they had stuck a needle into his thigh and injected some chemical that burned like fire all the way up through his body and then exploded inside his head.

The phrase they kept using was "arteriovenous malformation." He didn't know what it meant, but he knew by the way everybody acted that it was pretty serious.

Richard and his wife had sat and listened as Dr. Ducker explained that the AVM, as he called it, would get worse. It would expand further and bleed again and again. He would lose a little function with each hemorrhage, and perhaps he would be crippled.

Finally, the AVM would probably press against something that was attached to something that would kill him. Or it would bleed a lot, and *that* would kill him.

The alternative was to take it out.

Dr. Ducker had been straightforward. The operation was not without risk.

If Richard didn't want to chance it, Dr. Ducker wouldn't fault him for the choice. It might take many years for the AVM to disable and then kill him. The operation, on the other hand, posed a more immediate risk of death.

Richard had listened, but he had known all along what his choice would be. In fact, it wasn't really a choice. For one thing, there was the baby to think of.

If Richard died tomorrow, on Dr. Ducker's table, there would be insurance. If he lived and was slowly crippled by the malformation, there would be only hardship. He would be a liability to his family.

Now, the night before the operation, it would have been nice to have his wife here . . . but that was out of the question. She might go into labor at any moment, and what would happen if that rattletrap of a car broke down on the way here, or on the way back home? Suppose she was stranded beside the road, at night, and the baby started to come?

No, it was less of a worry to have her safe at home.

Richard closed his eyes and let the water beat against his face and plaster his hair back against his scalp.

What would it be like to die?

Richard didn't know, and he had never heard an explanation that satisfied him. The question made his empty stomach writhe.

He was scared, all right. He didn't deny it.

He bent over to turn up the hot water a little more.

There had been a time, not many years ago, when the fear would have been accompanied by the craving for heroin. Heroin could change the world around him, make it less frightening. But now he was older, wiser, stronger. If nothing else, he had accomplished that. If he died tomorrow, it would not be of an overdose, it would not be in some fleabag hotel, it would not be in filth.

The danger was real, but the fear was only chemicals. Like heroin, or alcohol, or filth, it could be endured. The fear was natural, normal. Let it come.

The water was hot now, right at the threshold of pain, and clouds of steam boiled along the bathroom ceiling. The soggy soap lathered easily on his hot skin, and the water washed away the suds.

He could die. He could be made stupid. He could wake up and be somebody else.

Richard wondered how it would feel to be someone else in his body. He probably wouldn't know the difference. That gave him the creeps. It would be a shame for the baby to have a dead father, but it would be more of a shame for him to have a stupid one. Death was definitely preferable.

He had tried to tell Dr. Ducker that. He'd tried to explain that life was important, but normalcy was everything. The words hadn't come out well, and Richard didn't know whether the surgeon had understood what he'd been trying to communicate.

Having fresh soap was nice.

His wife had brought it to him, this afternoon. It was a small thing, but it was thoughtful, the kind of thoughtfulness Richard appreciated. Later, after his wife left, a nurse had come in with three extra towels. They were brand-new, and fluffy white. That, Richard assumed, was also his wife's doing.

He missed her tonight, but there would have been nothing she could have done if she had stayed. The minutes had to pass, that was all. When enough minutes had passed, it would be over.

He turned off the water and the noise vanished.

Richard brushed most of the droplets from his body with the edge of his hand, then reached for the towel. He dried himself, caressingly. There was no luxury like a brand-new towel.

If fear was a chemical that welled up out of the deep brain, then courage was one you made yourself, on purpose, somewhere in the cortex.

For a while he lay on his bed in his pajamas, hands behind his head, staring at the ceiling.

He remembered the schizophrenic, that night, before the AVM had bled.

I believe in Lord Jehovah God.

Richard's words were too soft for anyone to hear but him. They didn't sound as silly as he thought they would.

He tried to remember the Sunday school lessons, as a child, in the old brick church. Was it Nazarene? Or was it Baptist? He couldn't remember. It was so long ago.

But he remembered singing a song.

Jesus loves me.

Richard hummed, softly, then recited, from deep in his memory.

The Lord is my shepherd, I shall not want; He maketh me to lie down in green pastures; He restoreth . . .

"Richard?"

Richard jumped. He hadn't heard the nurse come in.

She smiled at him and selected a little paper cup from a tray of drugs. She put the cup on the night table.

A sleeping pill, she said.

"I don't need a sleeping pill."

That's fine, she said. He didn't need to take it, if he didn't want to, but she'd leave it anyway. That way he could change his mind later.

When she left, Richard tried to fix his mind on God again, but the spell was broken. The feeling wouldn't come back.

The minutes were very real, and they passed very slowly, but Richard had dealt with minutes before. For a while, he scrutinized the landscape of the ceiling, which was white acoustic tile punctuated with holes. The holes were placed in such a way as to appear random, except, if you looked closely, there was a repeating pattern.

Later, he browsed through a newsmagazine. But newsmagazines didn't pass the minutes well. Richard, at the moment, was profoundly disinterested in Angola.

The baby would be a boy.

Or, alternatively, a girl.

Life was lived on a scale of minutes, right now, tonight, immediately, minutes that passed in various ways, one after another, with a flash of memory, followed by a moment of understanding, then an instant of terror, and the voice of his mother calling, Richard, Richard, Richard . . . or maybe some other name.

Eventually Richard sat up, swung his feet over the edge of the bed and slipped them into the still wet shower shoes. Picking up a clean, brand-new towel, he walked into the bathroom and closed the door.

A shower was a little thing, a thing few people considered.

One of Richard's big complaints about public housing, when it came down to what really mattered, was that there was never enough hot water. If he stood in a hot shower very long at home, it would suddenly turn cold. Richard had learned to tolerate lukewarm water, sacrificing the heat in the interest of more time in the shower.

But this shower was fed by the hospital's huge boilers, and Richard could use as much hot water as he wanted. He made the spray as hot as he could stand it, stepped under the shower head and waited. When his nervous system adjusted, he turned the hot water up some more.

It pounded down on his glistening skin and crashed against the tile wall. Drops of steam condensed on the mirror and ran down, leaving wet streaks on the foggy surface.

Richard stood in the scalding torrent, lathering and rinsing, oblivious to the passing of minutes, the Great Questions of life and death drowned out by the splashing roar of water.

CHAPTER
TWENTY-FOUR

WHEN GEORGE SAMARAS HAD FINALLY SATISFIED HIS STUBBORN computers, he had something he could be proud of. It was a fine enough creation, in fact, to deserve a name.

The engineers discussed the matter and several of them suggested Phoenix, after the legendary bird that rose anew from its own ashes. The other suggestion was Capricorn, the constellation that sits exactly opposite Cancer in the zodiac. George thought the symbolism of the latter one was more positive, and besides, he was a Capricorn himself. Since the deciding vote was his, Capricorn it became.

He and Michael tried it first on a cat. Michael did the surgery to implant the rod-like antenna, and George stood over Capricorn and watched the flashing lights. He didn't have much else to do.

The four computers consulted one another, noted minuscule changes in thermometer readings, and adjusted the microwave power accordingly. In the cat's brain, the temperature around the probe stayed rock-steady, one hundred and thirteen degrees Fahrenheit.

Periodically, the computer took time out to flash a reassuring message on the screen. All was well, the message said. Perfect.

George watched with pride as Capricorn worked. The microwave generator, monitored by the fabulous fail-safe, error-checking computer, was a beautiful example of what the new science of bioengineering could produce. It was a device that took ordinary sixty-cycle electricity out of a standard grounded wall plug and turned it into a treatment for cancer.

Later, Capricorn spewed out long strips of paper, filled with data and graphs that documented the treatment in extravagant detail.

When the first cat experiment worked so well, they almost immediately tried another. It, too, was perfect.

Dr. Salcman also admired Capricorn. It was even portable. Everything was built into a desk, which had wheels. No more huge racks of heavy equipment that swayed alarmingly as they were trundled along on appliance dollies. Dr. Salcman also appreciated the fact that Capricorn had much less surface for germs to hide on.

Another cat. Perfect. Another cat. Perfect.

Finally, they were ready.

Dr. Salcman scheduled Tony Mastrostephano for surgery. The morning before the chosen day, the neurosurgeon and the bioengineer did one last cat.

Perfect.

Dr. Salcman withdrew the probe from the cat's brain, gently, the way he would withdraw it from Tony Mastrostephano's. It slid out smoothly, harming nothing. The scientists wiped the antenna clean, detached it from Capricorn, and sent it over to surgery to be sterilized with ultraviolet light and poisonous gas.

That afternoon, they wheeled Capricorn over to the hospital and parked it in the storage room across from OR 11. George plugged it in and instructed it to test itself. For a moment the lights flashed and electrical charges surged through the computer cores.

Perfect, Capricorn soon reported. Everything was perfect.

The bioengineering group went off to the Campus Inn to celebrate. The next morning, Dr. Samaras and his assistant arrived at the hospital well before seven o'clock, changed into OR greens, and reconnoitered.

Kay Donnelly, the circulating nurse, and Doris Schwabland, the scrub nurse, were already busy arranging equipment and laying out instruments. A trainee was helping them. The anesthesiologist had an assistant this morning as well, and there would probably be spectators. There were always spectators when something unusual was happening.

The patient hadn't arrived yet.

Dr. Samaras decided to put Capricorn in a corner by the door of the autoclave room. It would be out of the way there. It wouldn't be needed until the operation was over, but Dr. Samaras wanted it to be in place to minimize confusion.

As the bioengineers moved Capricorn into the OR, Tony Mastrostephano arrived in the hallway on a gurney pushed by two nurses. The anesthesiologist and his assistant went out and chatted with Tony for a moment, reassuring him and making certain that he was appropriately groggy. Then they wheeled him back down the hallway to the X-ray room for one final, preoperative picture.

In the operating room a resident hung sixteen CAT scans and one standard X-ray on the lightboard behind the anesthesiologist's rack of machinery.

Dr. Samaras and his assistant pushed Capricorn to its chosen place, plugged it in and stood back to assess the arrangement. Perfect.

The morning did not begin so auspiciously for Dr. Salcman, however.

He had intended to use the laser to burn the tumor out of Tony Mastrostephano's brain. But the laser, Kay told him, was on the fritz. A red warning light was on and the controls didn't work.

Dr. Salcman worried with it for a few minutes. He checked its electrical supply, and assured himself that it had enough pressurized gas. Everything seemed in order, except that it wouldn't work. The neurosurgeon muttered something unflattering about the laser's designer.

So he was not in the best of moods as he entered the operating room. The first thing he noticed was that there were nearly a dozen people in there already.

That made Dr. Salcman slightly uneasy. Crowds meant germs, and germs meant infections. Things today seemed . . . well, less than perfect. The neurosurgeon walked through the OR to where Dr. Samaras was sitting at the Capricorn console. How was the machine? Dr. Salcman asked.

George glanced up and smiled. Fine. Perfect. What else?

He was about to run a test sequence, he told Dr. Salcman. After that, he had to go across town to Hopkins to give a talk. He would be back before the microwave antenna was implanted.

The neurosurgeon nodded and walked over to the X-ray board. Dr. Samaras directed his attention back to the console. He reached out and flipped the main switch. The electronic power meters lighted up with lines of zeros, and a tiny screen on the console slowly began to glow. Words appeared on it.

The bioengineer looked at the screen in disbelief.

The power, the fail-safe, error-checking computer was complaining in terse computerese, was unsatisfactory.

George stared, open-mouthed, at the message. What did it mean, there was no electricity?

The scientist's eyes immediately went to the power cord. It was plugged into the wall socket, all right. Of course it was. If Capricorn wasn't plugged in, it wouldn't have the energy to light up the screen and complain that it had no power.

He stared at the screen. "I don't believe this. Michael, come look at this."

Dr. Salcman walked over from the X-ray viewing board.

"This is crazy," Dr. Samaras said. "I'm getting a power status error. It's not possible, but there it is."

"Can you fix it?" the surgeon asked.

"I dunno," said the scientist, staring at the console. "Give me half an hour."

Dr. Salcman walked back to the X-ray board.

"I think I'm going to be sick," he said, to no one in particular.

When the anesthesiologists wheeled Tony into the operating room, Dr. Samaras was sitting at Capricorn, frowning and punching in commands. Every command produced the same response. Capricorn demanded electricity.

Dr. Salcman helped his patient move from the gurney onto the operating table. As soon as the patient was on his back, Kay Donnelly moved in and buckled a wide strap across his stomach.

"Everything is going to be just fine," Dr. Salcman told Tony. Tony grinned up at him, drunkenly.

"I'm going to lick this thing," he said, extending his left arm for the anesthesiologist.

Tony's right hand lay across his chest. Dr. Salcman put his palm over it and squeezed.

At the Capricorn console, a few feet away, George Samaras tried to coax the machine into doing something, anything. But every command received an identical reply. Give me electricity, Capricorn demanded. George shook his head, bewildered.

"I don't understand it," he said to himself, again and again. "I just don't understand it."

His eyes went back to the receptacle. It had two sockets. Capricorn was plugged into one of them. The other one was empty. Dr. Samaras got down on his knees in front of the receptacle.

There was a red dot on the receptacle plate. That meant it was connected to the emergency generators. Operating rooms couldn't afford to have power failures, and they didn't.

Dr. Samaras pulled out the plug and inserted it into the other socket. He got up, went back to the console, and turned it on.

No, said the fail-safe, error-checking computer.

Dr. Samaras looked one more time at the wall receptacle, then his eyes moved back to Capricorn. They stayed there, staring, for a very long time.

He had designed this accursed machine, supervised its construction, participated in its programming and debugging, and he damn sure hadn't made it capable of illogic. And yet it used the power he gave it to tell him to give it power.

He stood up, walked to a telephone in the autoclave room and started dialing. The folks over at Hopkins would have to listen to someone else today.

At 7:52 A.M. the anesthesiologist pushed the plunger on a syringe attached to Tony Mastrostephano's intravenous line. Tony's eyes rolled up and he went limp. A moment later, there was a plastic airway in his windpipe and the respirator was pumping measured bursts of oxygen into his lungs.

Two residents moved in. The razor blade made a rasping sound against the scalp as Tony's hair fell away. George Samaras was careful not to bump into them as he wheeled the Capricorn out across the hallway and into the storage room, where he could work without contaminating things.

Dr. Salcman was standing over the broken laser, hopelessly pushing buttons. He looked up as George went by with the desk, but he didn't say anything.

In a few minutes, having again given up on the laser, Dr. Salcman re-entered the OR.

"We'll do it anyway," he said, pulling a surgical mask over his nose and mouth. "If they don't have the system fixed by the time we're done, we'll plant the antenna anyway. Then we'll be ready if they get it working again."

Tony's shaved head gleamed in the bright OR lights. The whiteness vanished as the junior resident began scrubbing the scalp with dark-brown antiseptic.

Dr. Salcman looked up when Dr. Samaras stuck his head in the door.

"Michael, I'm up," the bioengineer said. "It works fine across the hall. I don't know what it is about this room."

Dr. Samaras disappeared back into the hallway and Dr. Salcman shifted his attention and stared thoughtfully at Tony's scalp.

"Anybody taking bets?" he finally asked. He got no answer.

The two residents covered Tony with green surgical drapes, until all that showed of him was a six-inch square of bare scalp. The scar from the first operation was clearly visible.

"The trouble with computers," Dr. Salcman mused, "is that they're not reliable. Any little thing can kill them. The human brain has circuits failing all the time, but it's got so much redundancy that it keeps right on working. Now *that's* sophistication."

At exactly 8:40, the chief resident's scalpel pressed against the exposed scalp. Blood welled up, and the junior resident stepped forward with the bipolar tweezers.

Dr. Salcman stood, watching the residents, talking to them.

"The microwave generator has four computers in it," he said, "and you can't get a committee of four to agree on anything."

"Scalp clips, please," the chief resident said. Quickly, he and his assistant worked to stanch the flow of blood and pull the scalp back across the side of the head.

"The only instruments a surgeon can really trust," Dr. Salcman went on, flexing his fingers, "are the ones he carries around with him all the time."

Across the hall, Dr. Samaras sat and looked at Capricorn. Everything was perfect. Whatever the problem was, it wasn't any more. But why?

What had he done wrong?

In the OR, the resident pulled the scalp back, revealing the bone. Dr. Salcman peered over the residents' shoulders at the top of Tony Mastrostephano's skull. It was easy to see where the Pennsylvania surgeon had opened Tony's head during the first operation. There was a four-inch rectangle of bone that hadn't quite healed back in.

Bone scar had sealed the flap along three edges, but the yellowish-white tumor protruded through the fourth. The two residents stopped working for a moment to look at the deadly tissue. Dr. Salcman shook his head, sadly.

"Take a specimen of that for pathology," he ordered. The chief resident sliced a small piece free with his scalpel, and handed it to the scrub nurse.

With Dr. Salcman supervising, the two residents proceeded to re-remove the bone flap. The air drill whined loudly, echoing off the tile walls.

Dr. Salcman watched, content. His part of the day, at least, was going well. He didn't like to take out a tumor with the suction tool— not after he'd paid good money for a laser. He'd rather use the laser, but he didn't need it. So that part would go all right.

Soon the bone flap was free. Doris took it in her rubber-gloved hand and placed it in a bowl of fluid beside her instrument tray.

Now Dr. Salcman and the two residents examined the dura. Normally, the leathery covering of the brain was milky-white, but in this case it was scarred and discolored. It had been breached in several places by the growing tumor.

The surgical pathologist opened the door of the operating room, paused a moment, and walked over to the X-ray board. He looked at the CAT scans for a moment, then shook his head.

"Glioblastoma multiforme," he announced, and left.

Dr. Salcman looked back at the surgical field. The residents had parted the dura and were beginning to dissect away the cancer. It looked as if it had grown deep into Tony Mastrostephano's right temporal lobe.

It was time to scrub.

On his way to the deepsink, Dr. Salcman paused to stick his head into the storage room. George Samaras was sitting in front of the machine, making it test itself again and again and again. Each time the answer was the same.

Everything was fine, Capricorn reported. The fail-safe, error-checking computer was working fine. The three other computers were working fine. The electricity was fine. No problems at all.

"What was wrong with it?" Dr. Salcman asked.

"You tell me," the bioengineer replied.

Shaking his head, Dr. Salcman turned and headed for the scrub sink.

In the storage room, Capricorn finished its self-diagnosis, printed the results, then helpfully added a dotted line and the notation, "Please tear here."

Outside, in front of the deepsink, Michael Salcman stepped on the soap switch. As he washed, suds crawled up his arm. Wash. Rinse. Wash. Rinse. A three-dimensional image of the brain floated through his consciousness.

He would go in from the top right, today.

The map rotated in his mind.

The scrub done, Dr. Salcman backed through the operating room doors, holding his dripping hands in front of his body. He dried them on a sterile towel and allowed Doris to wrap him in a green gown. She held out his rubber gloves by their cuffs, and he plunged his fingers into them.

Ready to work, he moved over to the patient. The junior resident stepped aside for him.

The dura had been pulled away, exposing the ugly tumor. It reminded him again what a depressing disease glioblastoma multiforme was.

Just five months before, a neurosurgeon with a laser had opened this skull and burned out every bit of tumor he could see. Now the cancer had already eaten further into the brain and added enough bulk to fill the surgical hole and force its way out through the healing dura. This, in the face of X-ray treatments and chemotherapy.

Dr. Salcman supervised, ready to step in, as the more junior of the two residents teased at the tumor. The operating microscope remained in its swung-back position, unused.

In the natural hierarchy of the operating room, the junior man was doing the least critical work. He removed the skull flap, opened the dura, and dissected away chunks of tumor with tweezers and the suction probe.

Now, with a sizeable hole cleared, the operation began to approach the stage where normal tissue might be encountered. When it was, it must not be damaged. Tony didn't have much left that he could afford to lose. So the chief resident took over.

He stripped away still more tumor from the edges of the cavity, gently, gently, a millimeter at a time, eyes focused on the tip of the suction probe, alert for the glistening white color which, in this part of the brain, would signify normal tissue.

But it was Dr. Salcman, and not the residents, who saw the first glimmer of white.

Stop, he said. The chief resident stopped instantly.

The operation was suspended while Dr. Salcman, the scrub nurse, and the junior resident draped the microscope in clear, sterile plastic. The chief resident backed away from the incision, and, holding his gloved hands in front of him, arched his spine backward and flexed his shoulders.

When the microscope was in place, the chief resident moved back in and fitted his face against the twin eyepieces. With a gloved finger, he manipulated a series of buttons. The focus changed, and changed again. Not yet satisfied, he altered the angle slightly. He had operated under Dr. Salcman's tutelage many times, and he handled the microscope expertly.

The circulating nurse turned a knob and the overhead lights dimmed, then went out. At the far end of the operating room, the color television monitor flickered and the screen filled with a blur of yellow, red and white.

The chief resident pressed another button and suddenly the picture leaped into sharp focus. The landscape was tortured and discolored.

The chief resident called for a microsucker, and the second phase of the operation got under way.

Across the hall, George had been joined by the rest of his engineering team. Now the various engineers were all standing around, trying to imagine what could make a machine use electrical impulses to tell you it wanted electricity.

Dr. Samaras described the problem to them again, as clearly as he could remember it. The engineers would have been more helpful if he could have made the Capricorn repeat its error, but he couldn't. Every time he turned it on, it worked fine.

In Operating Room Eleven, the removal of Tony Mastrostephano's tumor proceeded according to plan. Slowly, painstakingly, the chief resident whittled away at the growth, enlarging the hole. Dr. Salcman assisted from the side microscope, lecturing on the fine points of tumor removal. The junior resident and several visitors stood and watched the television monitor.

On the other side of the patient's body, the anesthesiologist's assistant watched the dials and meters. The heartbeat was steady, seventy-two beats a minute.

"Irrigation," the resident said, and the nurse handed him a small syringe filled with sterile water. The water flooded across the microscopic field and vanished into the mouth of the sucker.

Suction. Irrigation. Suction. Irrigation.

Finally the hole had enlarged dramatically, and there were traces of healthy tissue everywhere. Then the chief resident stepped to the side 'scope and Dr. Salcman took over.

Suction. Irrigation. Suction. Irrigation.

Slowly, methodically, Dr. Salcman whittled away at the sickly tissue.

Shortly before noon, the operating room door swung open and George Samaras and three assistants, all dressed in scrub suits, wheeled Capricorn back inside. The circulating nurse threw a green sterile drape over the machine before it came near the patient.

When the machine was parked in the same corner as before, the engineers clustered around it and reattached its various coaxial cables. Finally, one of them kneeled and plugged the power cord back into the receptacle.

Nearby, yet far away, Dr. Salcman stared through the microscope at one remaining speck of tumor. It was attached to the motor cortex and Dr. Salcman was frankly afraid to touch it. What point would there be in all this, if Tony was forced to live his last days as a cripple?

In theory at least, Dr. Salcman decided, the microwave treatments might take care of it.

"We're going to put the antenna into the superior vent of the temporal lobe," the neurosurgeon announced to the room at large. "It's gonna go right along the Sylvian fissure."

Doris, the scrub nurse, carefully unwound the coiled wires that trailed from the slender microwave antenna. She handed the antenna to Dr. Salcman, who held it up so that the residents could see that it was marked, like a ruler, in centimeter increments.

Then he laid it in place in Tony's brain and explained that, to be positioned the way he wanted it to be, it would have to be inserted six centimeters.

It couldn't be left in place now, of course. There was nothing to hold it in place. It would have to be inserted later, at just this precise angle, through the scalp and skull.

First, the dura would have to be stitched back up.

A few feet away, George Samaras flipped on Capricorn's master power switch. Its lights flickered, the screen glowed, and the fail-safe, error-checking computer demanded electricity.

Dr. Samaras stared at the machine, a look of utter hopelessness on his face.

The engineers stood in a group around the equipment, talking in low whispers. It wasn't logical for a computer to work in one room but not another. Not logical at all.

Dr. Salcman stood with them for a few minutes. Then, sighing, he walked away.

His part of it, at least, had been a perfectly successful operation. Even without the microwave, the operation might give Tony Mastrostephano another year of useful life. It would probably take that long for the tumor to refill the cavity. Dr. Salcman had done his job, and done it well. Now it was George's turn . . . maybe.

The residents began trying to stitch the dura, leaving a hole for the antenna shaft. The work went slowly, very slowly. The dura was so badly eroded by the cancer, drugs and radiation therapy that the stitches tended to tear loose. Patiently, the residents put them back.

The engineers stood and thought.

"Maybe the circuit's overloaded," suggested one. "We could turn everything off and see if that works."

The anesthesiologist's assistant, overhearing the proposition, straightened up suddenly. "Oh, goody," he exclaimed, his voice thick with sarcasm. "Let's turn off the respirator first."

The engineers glanced at one another and lowered their voices.

A few minutes later, one of them crawled under Capricorn with a test probe. He lay on his back, his feet sticking out, while he tested the circuits.

Dr. Samaras bent over the top of the console, staring at a portable voltmeter.

Under the operating lights, the chief resident used a small power drill to bore a hole in the skull flap, and made a matching hole in the scalp flap. Then, carefully, the surgeons lowered the whole thing over the incision.

All the holes lined up perfectly. Dr. Salcman threaded the antenna through them without difficulty.

"Look, George," Dr. Salcman said, delight in his voice. "It's a perfect match." But Dr. Samaras wasn't listening.

"I'm reading split ground now," said the man under the desk. Dr. Samaras frowned down at the voltmeter. Everything seemed to be perfect at his end, too, except that nothing worked.

Dr. Salcman bent over Tony's head, the scalp and bone flaps skewered by the antenna and cradled in his right hand. Slowly, he lowered the flaps over the hole. Everything fit perfectly. The chief resident quickly wired the skull flap in place, threading the wire through small holes he'd drilled before.

Dr. Salcman checked the markings on the probe, and subtracted the thickness of scalp and skull. The tip was exactly six centimeters into the brain. Perfect.

The engineers clustered around Capricorn.

"It's got to be the power line," Dr. Samaras' chief assistant finally said, in exasperation. "It can't be anything else. Let's get an extension cord and plug it in someplace else."

Dr. Salcman held the antenna in place while the chief resident wove a purse-string suture around the antenna probe and pulled it tight. Carefully, Dr. Salcman let go. The probe stayed in place.

Meanwhile Kay, the circulating nurse, had located a heavy-duty extension cord and given it to Dr. Samaras. "How about the autoclave room?" she asked, pointing to a receptacle around the corner. Dr. Samaras quickly plugged it in.

Dr. Salcman stepped away from the operating lights and let the junior resident take over to stitch down the scalp. The scrub nurse handed him a curved needle threaded with black silk thread. Dr. Salcman stood looking over the young man's shoulder, watching him work.

Dr. Samaras sat down at Capricorn's console and flipped the switch.

Perfect, the computer reported, instantly.

Perfect.

George stared at the machine, and then at the operating room wall plug.

He got up, walked to the plug he had been using all morning, kneeled, and pushed the voltmeter probe into one of the socket's openings. Frowning, he withdrew it and reinserted it into an adjacent hole.

Then, with elaborate slowness, he rose and wrapped the leads around the voltmeter.

"I would like to announce," he said loudly, "that there is nothing wrong with my machine. There never was. It's your power supply."

A few minutes later the electricity flowed through the microwave generator and into the antenna in Tony's head. The temperature rose quickly to one hundred and thirteen degrees Fahrenheit, and hung there steady, steady, rock-steady.

The first treatment lasted for precisely fifteen minutes.

It was perfect.

TWENTY-FIVE

EARLY THE MORNING OF JOE'S OPERATION A NURSE CAME IN AND GAVE him a shot of something that was supposed to make his mouth dry and his head woozy. It made his mouth dry, all right, but he was wide-awake and alert when they came for him with the gurney.

As they wheeled him down the hallway to an elevator Joe stared at the passing ceiling. They always took you down the hallway head-first, for some reason, and that was an interesting angle from which to view the world. Everybody towered above him in the elevator. Then he was in a seventh-floor hallway, and he heard the pneumatic doors open up ahead of him.

The only thing to do was be cool.

They parked him for a while in a tiny room next to the OR. He could see the shiny metal table and the overhead lights through an open door.

A lot of people introduced themselves to him and fussed around the gurney. The anesthesiologist hung a bottle of clear liquid over Joe's head and stuck a needle into his arm. The fellow was very expert: It didn't hurt much. Or maybe it was just that Joe was finally getting used to needles.

After they got the clear liquid dripping into his body through the IV line, they attached a stethoscope thing to his heart. It was attached to an amplifier. Joe listened to the liquid sound, ka-GLUP, ka-GLUP, ka-GLUP, like a washing machine with a load of towels. It was always interesting to hear the sound of your own heartbeat. For a while, curiosity helped Joe remain calm.

The anesthesiologist filled a small hypodermic syringe. He held it up and pressed the plunger until a little of its contents squirted out into the air, and then he pressed the needle against the plastic IV line. Joe saw the plunger move, and waited for the drug to take possession of his brain.

Faces swam slowly across his mind.

They all had masks on. He was the only one in the room who didn't have a mask.

Twenty seconds later, a respirator was breathing for him.

It was 8:10 A.M. The anesthesiologist noted the onset of unconsciousness in his notebook. The operating crew knew precisely what to do. As soon as Joe was obviously unconscious everyone who wasn't otherwise occupied converged to set up the Mayfield clamp. It took the anesthesiologist, his assistant, two residents and the circulating nurse to hold the wobbly structure until its joints could be tightened.

For the next few minutes the OR team moved about rapidly but quietly in the small room, arranging instruments, arranging equipment, arranging Joe. Soon two junior men prepared to shave off the stubble of hair Joe had spent the summer growing.

The chief resident told them to go very easy over the site of the old incision. He pointed to the soft bulge that protruded from the base of the skull, where the surgeons had made a hole in the skull before. They hadn't replaced the bone—the hole was tucked under the back of the head, protected by the big neck muscles. Besides, in a situation where the tumor regrows explosively, the hole allows for some expansion.

The resident touched the soft bulge. It almost jiggled to the touch. Something had grown in there and pushed out through the hole.

When they had stripped Joe of his sparse hair, the residents wiped the scalp dry. Then, touching lengths of masking tape to the skin, they removed stray hairs. Surgeons hated hair. It crawled with bacteria.

Once Joe's head was shaved, the team sat him up, bent his neck and held him steady as the Mayfield clamp bit through his scalp. Soon he hung from the clamp. He looked, from his attitude, as though he had just dozed off in a mathematics class and half-slumped down onto his desk, head forward and turned slightly to the right.

An assistant turned a crank under the table until it was low enough so the bulge behind Joe's left ear was at shoulder height. The chief resident shook his head. No. Wrong. The team steadied Joe again while the chief loosened the clamp to make an adjustment. Then another adjustment. A little more to the left, and then up.

It took several minutes to get Joe arranged just right beneath the operating room lights.

The microscope hung from the ceiling on a swing-away arm. The monitor was on, and as the residents tinkered with Joe and the clamp, his head occasionally swam into view on the overhead screen. The shaved landscape of his scalp was punctuated only by the thin rivulets of congealed blood where the Mayfield tongs pierced the skin.

The residents covered their patient with layer after layer of green cloth. By 9:30, the only visible part of Joe was a square of skin on the back of his head. In the center of it was a soft, ominous bulge.

Joe Trott was no longer Joe Trott. He was a piece of anatomical topography, a problem, a challenge, a surgical field.

Dr. Donlin Long entered the room unobtrusively, as the preparations drew to a close. He stood for a few minutes, watching, his back straight, his hands clasped behind his head. It was a relaxing position. The upcoming procedure, he knew, could turn into one of those long, long days.

The bulge at the back of Joe's neck—that was a real worry. It might be full of tumor, or swollen cerebellum, or fluid under pressure. Dr. Long hoped it was just fluid. But whatever it was, if he opened it incorrectly something might happen, pressures might change suddenly inside the brain, something might shift slightly, and Joe would die.

The neurosurgeon reviewed his tactics again, briefly, in his mind. The bulge was only the first of many somethings that might happen today.

It might be cancer. There were rare cases of benign acoustic tumors turning malignant. In Joe's case the regrowth had been breathtaking. If the tumor had turned malignant, Joe would probably die within a few months anyway. Dr. Long would just debulk it again and get out. What was the purpose of doing so much, and making the patient so sick, if he was going to die soon anyway?

Assuming the tumor was technically benign, the neurosurgeon reflected, it was certainly . . . aggressive. It had probably taken fifteen years or more for it to grow the first time. He and Dr. Murray had taken out, say, ninety percent. And in just five months, it had surpassed its former size and invaded Joe's posterior fossa with a vengeance.

Now, he was certain, the tumor would be stuck to every important artery and nerve in the posterior fossa. If he accidentally cut a nerve that ran through the tumor, Joe's face could be paralyzed, or he'd never swallow normally, or one eye would never work right—but at least he would be alive. Sever an artery accidentally and it's Big Red.

And then there was the brain stem. The pilot light. Bump the brain stem, or damage a tiny artery leading to it, and something profound might happen to the connection between Joe's brain and soul, and he would live on, and on, and on . . . but never wake up.

The tumor would be stuck tight to the brain stem. Dr. Long knew, just knew, it would be.

He moved up to examine the bulge again, more closely. If it was swollen cerebellum, he'd have to work around it somehow. Dr. Murray had had to cut some of the cerebellum out before, to relieve pressure, and Joe could not afford to lose any more. It would be easier, much easier, if the bulge were tumor tissue, which he could cut away, or a fluid buildup, which he could drain.

Dr. Long turned to his chief resident and told him to put a tap into Joe's high ventricles. The tap could help determine the pressure inside the head and, if an internal shift seemed imminent, the tap could be used to drain fluid and equalize pressures.

"And hook up the Cavitron," the chief of neurosurgery added. "We're going to need it early."

While Dr. Long went outside to scrub, the chief resident changed the drapes to expose the top of Joe's skull. Then, assisted by a more junior resident, he made a small incision in the scalp. After the bleeding was stopped, a tiny retractor stretched the scalp open and held it there, exposing the white bone below.

"Craniotome," said the chief resident.

Before he handed it to him, the scrub nurse pressed the trigger once, just testing.

Zhoop.

The chief resident took the tool, pressed the bit against the skull, adjusted his body until he found a comfortable position, and touched the button.

Zhoop, zhoooooop, zhooooooooooooooooooooooo . . .

The resident rocked the drill back and forth to free the bit, and absently handed it back to the scrub nurse.

Outside, Dr. Long stood at the deepsink, washing his hands and thinking ahead. One thing was certain. The Cavitron would be a tremendous help today. If he'd had the Cavitron, he might have been able to get the whole tumor out of Joe's head the first time around.

The Cavitron was similar to the laser, in the sense that both of them were designed to remove tumor tissue. But they used different means to that end, and each had its advantages and disadvantages. The laser was wonderful for delicate work, like around the edge of a glioblastoma tumor. But Dr. Long considered the Cavitron more efficient for removing tough bulky tumors from dangerous places like the posterior fossa.

The Cavitron apparatus consisted of a cart of electronic equipment attached by wires and tubes to an instrument that resembled a long, fat pencil. The small needle protruding from the sharp end vibrated at such high speed that it disintegrated and liquefied the cells it touched. A fine spray of sterile water from around the needle washed away the debris. Suction ports, also on the tip, swept away the water and the tumor-cell puree.

With the Cavitron you still had to touch the brain, but only lightly. And the Cavitron was a mechanical gizmo at bottom, less vulnerable to electronic gremlins. Dr. Long had heard some bad reports about the laser's reliability.

Also, it was easy to burn through a blood vessel with a laser. But the rubbery vessels resisted the vibrations of the Cavitron. Of course, the Cavitron would probably go right through the brain stem.

Dr. Long fervently hoped he would never find out.

Neurosurgery was a profession requiring attention to detail, and it carried with it an attendant risk. The neurosurgeon's nightmare was of focusing on the trees and getting lost in the forest.

"It's a sinking feeling," Donlin Long had once confided, "when you have gotten yourself disoriented because you are concentrating on some abnormality . . ."

He had hesitated, groping for words, trying to describe the un-thinkable.

". . . you are working away on it when you suddenly discover . . . a very strong possibility . . . of being somewhere you have no business being.

"You suddenly discover . . . that you think . . .

". . . you are inside the brain stem, or . . . you have dissected through the optic nerve. There are a number of places where that can happen, and the more experienced you get, the less likely it is to happen, but there is no feeling like . . . suddenly recognizing where you are . . . and being immediately certain *you have no business being there.*"

And today, Joe Trott's tumor would have wrapped itself around the brain stem, the rising basilar artery and the cranial nerves. All of those things would be tubes of softness running through the firm tumor, and getting lost would be easy, so easy . . .

Dr. Long reviewed the topography of the posterior fossa, reminding himself of the exact location of the aye-ka, and the basilar. A three-dimensional mental map of the brain sorted itself through his neurons, and the image turned easily in his mind.

The approach would be from the back. For a change, right was right, left was left, up was up and down was down.

Dr. Long backed through the door of the operating room, hands dripping, shortly after the resident had finished drilling the burr hole. The scrub nurse turned his attention to Dr. Long, broke open a sterile pack and handed him a towel.

The chief neurosurgeon wrapped himself in a sterile gown and slipped on the rubber gloves.

The resident gazed down into the burr hole at the milky-white dura below. It bulged upward, but only slightly, which meant the pressure was high, but not too high. Soon Dr. Long was looking over his shoulder. He agreed.

The nurse handed the resident a long, sterile needle. For a moment, he held it poised, carefully. Its tip made a tiny dimple where it pressed against the dura. Then the resident moved his fingers and the needle slid slowly downward through the dura, into the brain. The resident's unblinking eyes fixed on the spot where the needle disappeared into the dura.

Suddenly, the tip of the probe entered the forward portion of Joe's right ventricle. Spinal fluid dribbled out the other end of the needle and the resident's fingers instantly ceased to move. That far, and no farther.

With a few deft stitches, the resident secured the drain in place and sutured the scalp around it. He screwed a metal cap over the outside end to cut off the flow of fluid. Now Dr. Long had a safety valve, an overflow drain and a pressure vent instantly available, just in case . . .

At 9:48, Dr. Long and the resident stood looking at the big soft bulge on the back of Joe's head. Finally, Dr. Long drew his finger along the back of the head and over the bulge. Then he stood back while the resident followed the imaginary line with the scalpel, parting the white flesh.

As the resident cut his way around three sides of what would become the scalp flap, Dr. Long came along behind him and placed the white plastic scalp clips along the incision to pinch off the flow of blood.

As soon as they got started, it became unusually difficult to recognize things. The membranes and the muscles of the neck had regrown, welded together with scar tissue. Nothing looked like it did in the anatomy reference books. That was the special danger of doing second operations.

Dr. Long identified the landmarks deductively, remembering exactly what should be exactly where, even if it looked nothing like it should.

The flesh over the bump parted easily. Beneath it was a reddish membrane of some sort, and behind that . . . well, they would soon find out. Gingerly, Dr. Long reached out a gloved finger and tested the membrane. Soft, flexible, like a balloon with water in it.

"Is he changing at all?" Dr. Long asked, directing his voice at the anesthesiologist.

The anesthesiologist scanned his instruments again. The heartbeat was solid, seventy-five. The blood pressure was one twenty-five over eighty-five. "No change," he told the surgeon.

Dr. Long pushed a little harder with his fingertips. "Still no change? I'm compressing him a little bit."

"No change." The heartbeat was steady, seventy-five beats per minute. The heart-sound amplifier gurgled reassuringly, ka-GLUP, ka-GLUP.

The chief resident pushed red muscle tissue aside, exposing more and more of the unusual red membrane. Dr. Long stopped him, and they stood for a moment, watching the bulge. It sloshed and heaved with every heartbeat.

Liquid.

Every movement was slow and measured. The circulating nurse opened the sterile package, and the scrub nurse reached his gloved hand inside to withdraw the syringe. He handed it to Dr. Long, who stood for a moment, balancing the needle. Then slowly, ever so slowly, he pierced the membrane and then drew carefully on the plunger. The syringe filled with cloudy liquid.

The liquid was white, the neurosurgeon explained, because it was full of coagulated protein.

The membrane began to sag as the pressure was released. By 10:04, it had collapsed. Dr. Long took a deep breath. One problem down, many left to go. He stepped back to make room for the resident.

The younger man stepped forward and parted the membrane from bottom to top with a pair of surgical scissors. The drapes beneath Joe's neck turned dark and wet as more milky fluid ran out, flowed along the cloth, and splattered on the floor.

The two surgeons stared into the cavity that had held the liquid. It was the size of a hen's egg. It extended deep into the brain, and everywhere its walls were lined by a coating of alabaster-white protein. A lake of milky liquid still lay across the bottom, and dark veins snaked along the walls. An artery pounded, rhythmically.

The tumor capsule would be beyond the far wall.

Dr. Long turned to the scrub nurse. "Drape the 'scope for us while we're doing this," he said, "and turn on the Cavitron."

The clock said 10:11.

While the scrub nurse was busy arranging the clear plastic drape over the operating microscope, Dr. Long took his place at the instrument table and began handing instruments to the resident. The younger man washed the protein off the walls of the cave with a syringe of sterile water. He removed the remaining liquid with a sucker probe.

Dr. Long watched from the side, his hands near the instrument tray.

Even at that distance, he could see the scarring from the previous operation. Scar tissue was always tougher than normal tissue. It contorted the landscape, sometimes beyond recognition. Sometimes, in a second operation, there was so much scarring that you couldn't tell where tumor ended and normal brain began. In the posterior fossa, that could be deadly.

The scrub nurse swung the microscope into position. Dr. Long relinquished the instrument tray back to him, and stepped to the 'scope.

With his eyes firmly pressed to the lenses, Dr. Long's world narrowed. Details of the cave's back wall swam into focus on the monitor. The chief resident and the scrub nurse stood ready to hand him instruments, make adjustments, guide his hands and perform all the other helpful tasks that would allow him to keep his attention fixed on the deadly landscape.

Carefully, the surgeon peeled back the far wall of the cave and the ugly yellow tumor came into view. Somewhere, embedded in it, would be the basilar artery and the aye-ka. It would be stuck to the brain stem, too.

With the suction probe in his left hand and the bipolars in his right, Dr. Long gingerly explored the exposed surface of the tumor.

The first step in any operation like this was to reconnoiter and assess the tactical situation. There was a second purpose, too. In the process of exploring the face of the tumor, Dr. Long would define its boundaries, loosen them from the brain where he could, remember the places where he couldn't.

"Microdissector," Dr. Long said, eyes pressed to the lenses. He extended his right hand in the general direction of the scrub nurse. The nurse removed the bipolars from it, and replaced them with a long-handled probe with a tiny, blunt top. For several seconds, Dr. Long balanced it in his fingers, until he got it just right, then lowered it into the cave. The resident guided his hand until the probe heaved into view in the monitoring screen.

Gently, Dr. Long used the blunt instrument to poke and scrape at the face of the tumor. He could see where it adjoined what looked like normal tissue on both the right and the left. The tumor was stuck firmly to it.

The first thing to do was find something recognizable.

Dr. Long's first assault on the tumor was to try to peer over it. Perhaps the fifth cranial nerve, the one that serves the face, could be seen. The fifth nerve split into three trunks where it emerged from the brain stem: It could be easily recognized.

But, after working for several minutes, Dr. Long didn't find it. Presumably, it had been engulfed by the tumor, and was now somewhere inside. Too bad. If he could have found and freed the fifth nerve, he'd have been in a good position to find and free the other nerves.

Failing to find the fifth nerve, Dr. Long retreated and turned his attention to poking and probing along the demarcation line between tumor and normal brain to the right and left. If he could start teasing them apart, if he could find a plane . . . but he couldn't. The tumor was stuck tight. He didn't dare pull.

There was scar tissue everywhere. Dr. Long worked slowly, thoughtfully, constantly mindful of the danger of getting lost.

Finally, he stepped back from the microscope. "This isn't working," he announced. "Let's reposition and try to go underneath."

The resident helped him tilt the microscope to a new angle. Then they adjusted the operating table slightly, and Dr. Long once again fitted his eyes against the microscope. With the blunt dissector, he probed along the lower wall of the tumor.

Back and forth, gently, gently, irrigation, suction, cotton ball, irrigation, suction.

Nothing. Nothing came loose. Nothing was recognizable.

Now there was only one approach left, and that was straight through the tumor, not knowing where anything was. He would have to be careful. Odds were that there would be several of Joe's cranial nerves embedded inside the tumor. It would be a lot easier if he could see where they entered, but he'd have to do without that luxury.

"Microscissors," he said, holding out his hand. A moment later, the tiny shears appeared in the microscopic field. They jockeyed for position, touched the tumor capsule and snipped a hole in it. Slowly, deliberately, the scissors opened the front of the capsule. Beneath, its yellow tissue sparkled in the microscope's headlights.

When the tumor capsule was open all across its face, the scissors found and clipped loose a piece of it. Dr. Long lifted it out and gave it to the scrub nurse.

"Label this one 'cyst capsule,' " he said.

The scissors went back inside. This time, they clipped off a piece of the tumor itself.

". . . and this one," he said, handing it to the nurse, ". . . I want this one called 'cerebellopontine angle tumor: question malignancy.' "

The scrub nurse put the samples into vials, capped them and handed them to the circulating nurse. The circulating nurse labeled the vials and left to deliver them to the surgical pathologist.

Dr. Long directed his attention back to the tumor. He studied it for a few moments and then, working with extreme caution, he began sweeping the tip of the sucker back and forth across the tumor, searching for any break in the glistening yellow. The nerve sheaths would be white, not yellow. They would also be softer than the tumor tissue.

In a few minutes, a speck of white appeared. The instruments withdrew a millimeter, then advanced again, slowly. Dr. Long brushed it with the suction probe, nudged it with the bipolars.

It was definitely a nerve, but which one? Whichever one it was, it was far out of position.

Experimentally, he directed the sucker to the side of the nerve and eroded away some more tumor tissue.

It was probably the fifth nerve, the facial nerve. If it was inside the tumor, then so would the sixth, and very likely the third and fourth . . . it would be a very, very long day.

As he worked with the sucker, eroding the tissue from around the nerve, his confidence in his original identification grew steadily. Part of the nerve was buried only very shallowly in the tumor and he freed it. It led back over the top of the tumor, to the brain stem. The other end dived deep into the yellow tumor mass. That would have to wait.

Now he used the tweezer-like bipolars to tuck several tiny wads of moist cotton behind the fifth nerve, to cushion it and keep it from drying out, and to make it immediately recognizable.

Well. At least he had identified something.

He studied the wall of the tumor, frowning.

Irrigation. Suction. Bipolars.

As he eroded away the tumor, the sucker encountered occasional small arteries and veins. Sometimes Dr. Long saw them before they burst, and burned them shut before going farther. Other times, without warning, the field just turned red. Irrigation, suction, bipolars . . .

Zzzzzzzt.

". . . there!"

And the surgical advance moved on.

Another nerve emerged from the yellow mass. "I believe that's the seventh nerve," Dr. Long said to the resident, not taking his eyes from the microscope barrels.

Suction . . . irrigation . . . bipolars.

Slowly the second hand of the OR clock moved around again and again and again. The monitors beeped steadily, seventy-five beeps a minute. Ka-GLUP, ka-GLUP, ka-GLUP went the heart-sound amplifier. Atop the respirator, a circular bellows enclosed in a glass tube moved up and down, up and down, up and down.

Finally the seventh nerve, too, was freed, tucked aside, and cushioned with cotton.

At 11:50 the surgical pathologist stuck his head in the door.

"Dr. Long!" said the nurse, softly. Dr. Long stood back from the microscope. His eyes moved to the pathologist.

"Schwannoma," the man said. "It was similar to the material you removed during the first operation."

The pathologist disappeared and the door slowly closed behind him. Dr. Long stood beside the microscope, looking reflectively into the hole in Joe Trott's head and breathing a sigh of relief.

So it wasn't malignant.

It was still a huge, gristly, overgrown wart with a sticky membrane. It was a considerable enemy, but conquerable.

The heart monitor beeped steadily, seventy-five beats a minute.

Dr. Long studied the tumor under the microscope. "Okay," he finally said, taking a deep breath. "Cavitron please. Let's go for broke."

It took several minutes to arrange all the various wires and hoses attached to the Cavitron, but eventually Dr. Long stood at the microscope with the pointed wand in his right hand.

It was a very large instrument by neurosurgical standards, and it was certainly more awkward to use than a laser. Dr. Long tested several arm and body positions before he was comfortable enough to lower the wand into Joe's head. Finally, he pressed his eyes to the microscope.

"Cavitron on," he said quietly.

The chief resident stepped on a foot switch. There was a faint high-pitched whine, almost beyond the range of the human ear.

Under the microscope, the black tip of the Cavitron moved too fast for the eye to detect it, and appeared to be standing still. Tentatively, the instrument moved toward the tumor wall. It touched it, and moved, leaving behind a trench.

The tip repositioned, touched the center of the tumor, then touched again and again. A hole appeared in the tumor and steadily grew. Dr. Long paused frequently to examine the inner surface of the tumor for telltale flecks of white or gray.

An hour passed. The anesthesiologist sat motionless, surrounded by his instruments. The neurosurgeon spoke to the scrub nurse and the chief resident in short, clipped sentences. He found another nerve, extricated it, and tucked it aside. Then another. The hole in the tumor grew deeper, and the wall sometimes collapsed inward. With each touch of the Cavitron, the surgeon moved a little closer to the deep forbidding structures of the basilar artery and the brain stem.

If Joe's tumor had turned cancerous, Dr. Long certainly wouldn't have tried to strip it off the basilar, the big artery that rose from the spine and fed all the arteries of the cerebellum, including the aye-ka. The basilar also had tiny branches of its own that dove deep into the brain stem.

At the same time, the tumor capsule would be glued tightly to the basilar, and to the tiny little arteries that flowed out from it. To cure Joe, Dr. Long would have to strip the tumor capsule off, pull it . . . no, not pull it, of course. Tease at it, suggest . . . beg.

If the basilar should tear in the process, there would be an explosion of blood boiling up from below, and Joe . . .

Dr. Long would undertake the basilar problem first. He was fresher now than he would be later. It would take a while to get to it but, once the basilar was free of tumor, he could quit worrying about it.

Back and forth, back and forth, the tip of the Cavitron probe swept across the tumor tissue, liquefying it and sucking it away. Occasionally Dr. Long had to halt the march to burn a tiny bleeder closed. With the Cavitron, that was easy. The torn end of the bleeder got pulled instantly into the suction ports of the instrument, keeping the field clear of blood and stretching out the torn vessel. Dr. Long could reach in easily, catch its base between the tongs of the bipolars and burn it closed.

Eventually, the neurosurgeon could see the far wall of the tumor, a veil of tissue that jiggled and pulsed in syncopation with the heart monitor.

It was as he had feared. The membrane lay wrapped partially around the basilar and was stuck tightly to it. He could see it throbbing through the membrane.

Thoughtfully, the neurosurgeon withdrew the Cavitron and the bipolar tweezers from the hole, then stepped back from the micro-scope and sat down on a stool. He stared at the television monitor screen, flexing his hands, arms and shoulders as he thought. Except for the beep, beep, beep and the ka-GLUP, ka-GLUP, ka-GLUP, the room was silent.

"We've probably got seventy-five or eighty percent of the tumor out now," Dr. Long finally said. His voice was preoccupied and directed at no one in particular. "We're done . . . with the easy part."

Again and again he flexed his right hand. He wished the Cavitron were lighter.

Dr. Long's musings were interrupted by Dr. Michael Holliday, who specialized in ear, nose and throat surgery. Dr. Holliday stuck his head through the door and asked, cheerfully, "Are you ready for me yet?"

"We will be shortly," Dr. Long replied, moving back to the micro-scope.

The ENT man's role in the operation was to be relatively brief, but very important. The tumor, like most of its type, had actually sprouted from a location inside the bony canal that led from the ear to the floor of the cranium. If Dr. Long was going to get all the tumor, it would be necessary to drill out the bone at the mouth of the canal, en-larging it enough for the instruments to get in and work efficiently.

The procedure, like every other in the posterior fossa, had its risks. Right next to the ear canal was the jugular bulb, through which a big vessel carried spent blood from the brain down to the jugular vein. The hearing canal would have to be excavated with a tiny power drill. One slip and the jugular bulb next door would tear, and blood would fill the surgical cavity.

Some neurosurgeons did their own drilling, but Dr. Long preferred to leave that part to Dr. Holliday. The ENT surgeon worked in bone more often than Dr. Long did. And he knew the hearing canal's com-plex anatomy in more minute detail. As a fringe benefit, it meant Dr. Long could break for lunch while Dr. Holliday worked.

First, the neurosurgeon must clear the ear canal area of tumor. Dr. Long peered through the microscope, balancing the heavy instrument.

"Cavitron on."

Working quickly with a side-to-side motion, Dr. Long stripped away tumor tissue, following alongside the exposed seventh nerve, burrowing a second hole toward the ear canal.

Microscissors.

Blunt dissector.

Irrigation.

For a few minutes Dr. Holliday watched over Dr. Long's shoulder, then he left to scrub. By the time he returned, Dr. Long was standing back from the microscope, his gown and rubber gloves off, vigorously massaging his right arm.

After turning the operation over to the ENT expert, Dr. Long walked out into the hallway. A few minutes later, in the OR cafeteria line one floor above, he continued unconsciously flexing his tired right hand. The chief resident stood behind him.

There were only a few other people in the small cafeteria, all of them wearing OR greens. Dr. Long took his tray to the cashier, who quickly tallied up his Polish hot dog, potato chips and soda. Then he carried the food to an empty table.

As he ate, he planned, worried and repeatedly chastised himself aloud for holding the Cavitron probe too tightly. He knew he was holding it too tightly, and that was why his muscles were aching. But it was so much heavier than he was used to. He constantly forgot, and had to relax his grip.

Besides, the Cavitron still frightened him a little. The thing was making short work of the tumor, which was about the consistency of gristle. If the Cavitron went right through that, what would it do if it accidently touched a nerve or a piece of brain tissue? One slip, and Joe might disappear up the barrel of the probe.

Dr. Long shuddered at the thought. Better to hold on to the Cavitron a little too tightly. If he got tired, he could rest.

As for Joe . . . so far, so good. Of course, what had been accomplished so far was the easy part, if anything about this case could be called easy. The tumor was debulked now, for the most part. It was time to begin peeling its rind from the basilar and brain stem.

Dr. Long and the chief resident exchanged views on tactics, then ate in silence. Soon the resident rose and returned to the operating room. Dr. Long stopped by his office to see how many letters and phone calls had piled up during the morning.

It was slightly after 1:30 P.M. when Dr. Long, freshly scrubbed, entered the OR again. By that time, Dr. Holliday had finished drilling out the ear canal and was gathering up his tools. The neurosurgeon slipped into gown and gloves and took his place at the microscope.

Twice he repositioned the microscope, surveying the landmarks. The ivory-colored brain stem hung in the background, near the throbbing basilar. On the floor of Joe's skull, where the ENT man had chipped away the obscuring bone, Dr. Long could now see the jugular bulb, and the bit of tumor that was attached to it. The heart monitor beeped steadily, seventy-five beats a minute.

"Cavitron, please."

The machine's high-pitched whine filled the room as Dr. Long brushed the tip against the bit of tumor in the ear canal. In a matter of minutes it was gone.

Dr. Long shifted his attention to the jugular bulb. There was a patch of tumor stuck to it, too. It appeared to be stuck very tightly.

He considered his options for a moment. No, he would leave the jugular bulb until last. If the bulb tore open, he could probably save the situation by packing a fibrous, clot-inducing material around it. But if he did that, he'd have to get out fast. Best to leave the bulb until last; if he did have to beat a hasty retreat, he wouldn't leave the rest of the tumor in Joe's brain.

Dr. Long sincerely did not want to do this operation again.

Next . . . the basilar.

The chief resident helped Dr. Long redirect the microscope so that it pointed toward the center of Joe's head. As the image came into focus, Dr. Long could see the intact far wall of the tumor, heaving in perfect time with the basilar artery behind it.

Dr. Long had begun the operation searching for a separation plane, and there was none. Now he would have to make his own.

He held out his hand. "Microscissors."

A millimeter at a time, he snipped through the tumor capsule, well away from where it joined to the basilar. He tested with tweezers after each tiny cut, lifting, probing, nudging.

No one spoke. The loudest noise in the OR was the steady beep, beep, beep of the heart monitor.

The OR was cool, almost chilly, but as Dr. Long worked so close to the basilar, tiny beads of sweat appeared on his forehead. Millimeter by agonizing millimeter, he worked his way along the tumor capsule, snipping, probing, snipping, probing. Slowly, in the background, the brain stem appeared. It glistened in the lights. There was tumor stuck to it, too.

Slowly, slowly, a blunt instrument swam into view and, ever so lightly, touched the brain stem.

"Watch him," Dr. Long warned the anesthesiologist. "My right-hand retractor's on the brain stem. Tell me if he changes at all."

The heart beat steadily, ka-GLUP, ka-GLUP, ka-GLUP.

"Is he changing at all?"

"No. He's stable."

"I'm right on the basilar now."

Steady, seventy-five beats a minute.

With the probe, Dr. Long stroked the tumor capsule where it clung to the basilar. The capsule remained stuck. He stroked it again and again, until the motion began to reduce the yellow tissue to tatters. The basilar throbbed.

"The tumor is plastered right down the side of the basilar," Dr. Long told the operating room team, his eyes not moving from the microscope. "I'm taking it off a millimeter at a time, and I'm afraid that any time . . ."

Slowly, painstakingly, he nudged at the tumor, beckoned to it, urged it, worried at it, and, bit by bit, teased it free. The clock hands turned.

Gently, gently.

Nudge and probe.

Stroke.

Scissors, please.

Good. Microdissector.

The afternoon wore on and the tumor came to him, piece by tiny piece. The basilar throbbed under the lights. Slowly, tortuously, he stroked the capsule. Finally it sagged downward, away from the basilar.

"Oh," Dr. Long said, sudden relief in his voice, "it's starting to move. Oh, happy day!"

The anesthesiologist watched his dials. The heart beat steadily, seventy-five beats a minute, seventy-five beats a minute, perfectly.

With the dissector, Dr. Long probed for a moment at the loose end of tumor capsule. Where it attached to the basilar, there was a clear, clean, separation plane. Smile wrinkles appeared above the neurosurgeon's mask.

Carefully, Dr. Long put pressure, ever so slight a pressure, certainly not a pull, on the free end. A little more came loose. He stroked it, and the plane between the tumor and the capsule opened still farther. Within thirty minutes the lower half of the basilar was free of tumor.

As the capsule came free, it revealed the tiny branches of the artery.

"Wow!" the chief resident finally said from the side 'scope. "Look at them all!"

"Yeah," Dr. Long replied. "And any one of them can do him in."

He pointed the dissector at one small vessel in particular. A piece of tumor was still sticking to it.

"There's one we certainly don't want to lose," he said. "That's the aye-ka."

Dr. Long tucked a cotton ball behind the aye-ka, and, its location firmly established in his mind, he turned his attention back to the main tumor. He would face that problem later.

With the tumor capsule stripped from the lower half of the basilar, Dr. Long shifted the microscope to aim it at the upper half.

He pressed his eyes to the microscope and reached out the dissector, slowly, carefully . . .

And Joe jumped.

"HEY! WHOA!" Dr. Long shouted, jerking the instruments out of the hole as though he'd been shocked. "What happened?"

The neurosurgeon's head was away from the 'scope, his angry eyes focused on the anesthesiologist. The anesthesiologist, frantically filling a syringe, emitted a muffled, inaudible answer.

"Something happened," Dr. Long insisted, his voice sharp and imperial. "What was it? Did someone bump the table? Or did he move?"

Ka-GLUP, ka-GLUP, ka-GLUP.

Finally, the anesthesiologist spoke up. "He moved," he acknowledged, thrusting the needle into a plastic tube that led, under the layers of surgical drapes, to Joe's arm.

"I don't want him to move!"

Dr. Long took a deep breath and visibly relaxed.

It was an old, old problem. For the patient's safety, the anesthesiologist was motivated to use an absolute minimum of drugs. An over-generous use of anesthesia could burn a patient's brain out, which was why anesthesiologists paid such astonishing malpractice insurance premiums. The anesthesiologist was doing exactly what he was supposed to do.

But still . . .

What would happen if, at some critical moment, the patient moved, and the probe touched the brain stem a little too hard? A neurosurgeon's instant reaction to a movement by his patient is anger at the anesthesiologist.

"Look," Dr. Long said in a reasoning tone, "I don't want him to move. What I'm doing is sorta delicate. When this is all over and I look at him and say, 'Hello, Joe, how are you feeling?' he can move then. Not before then. Okay?"

The incident was over quickly, and Dr. Long's eyes were back at the lenses.

The separation plane seemed a tiny bit easier to establish on the upper portion of the tumor, or else Dr. Long was getting his second wind. Minutes passed. The wall clock crept past 4 P.M., but Dr. Long didn't notice.

The upper half of the basilar presented even more potentially deadly traps than had the lower. As he whittled away at the tumor attached to it, he assembled a mental picture of Joe's tumor and its character.

It was easily the biggest acoustic tumor Dr. Long had ever done—the biggest he'd ever seen, for that matter. It was, he suspected, even bigger than any in the literature. It had been large the first time, and it had grown back still larger. On the scale that governs the brain, it was huge, enormous, gigantic.

The thing had grown out of a speck of Schwann cells that had helped wrap part of the auditory nerve. Growing ever larger, it had oozed out toward the center of the head. It had wrapped around every blood vessel available, including the aye-ka. It had infiltrated itself around ten of Joe's twelve cranial nerves, nerves he used to focus his eyes, wet his lips, smile, talk, swallow . . .

Before the day was done, Dr. Long would have tinkered with all those things. He would have disturbed the nerves, tinkered with the brain stem, moved things around.

In Dr. Long's opinion, which was the one that counted, much of the trouble after Joe's first operation resulted from some well-meaning soul offering the lad a drink of water. Since Joe's swallowing nerves had been damaged, some of the water had run directly into Joe's lungs, causing a form of pneumonia.

This time, Dr. Long had given detailed, specific instructions to make sure the same thing didn't happen again. Now he reinforced those orders.

"Joe's going to be sick for a while," he said to the resident, not looking up. "I wouldn't let him eat for a long time."

"We'll keep the icebox locked," promised the chief resident, uncomfortably.

". . . for about a year," Dr. Long said, with a chuckle.

"Yes, sir."

When the basilar was stripped of tumor, the atmosphere in the OR became noticeably less tense.

Dr. Long readjusted the microscope and examined the brain stem. It was covered with tumor all the way from the very top of the posterior fossa down to the foramen magnum, where the stem narrowed and disappeared into the spine.

Dr. Long stuck out his hand for the dissector, and the scrub nurse supplied it.

The clock crept toward 5 P.M., seven hours into the operation.

Ka-GLUP, ka-GLUP, ka-GLUP, ka-GLUP, seventy-five times a minute.

Slowly, slowly, urging, coaxing, nudging, almost by force of will alone, Dr. Long separated the tumor capsule from the brain stem. Finding a cleavage plane, he followed it up, then down.

After a very long time, Dr. Long stepped back, working his arms and shoulders stiffly. In fifteen years as a neurosurgeon, Dr. Long had learned to ignore his aching muscles, to keep working for hours, oblivious of the pain and the passage of time. When he became cramped, he turned his attention away from the brain stem problem. He stripped the tumor from the aye-ka. By comparison, the procedure was almost relaxing. He freed the eleventh and twelfth nerves, and then the third, fourth, fifth, and sixth.

Finally, after four uninterrupted hours of operating, a tortured muscle failed to obey his command. An instrument clicked lightly against a retractor.

Abruptly, Dr. Long stood up.

"Take the main 'scope," he told the resident. He indicated a tag of tumor that still clung to the brain stem.

"See if you can take that off, while I rest my shoulder and see if I can get some movement back in my right hand."

While the chief resident whittled at the tumor Dr. Long collapsed heavily on a stool, rubbed his arms and flexed his fingers.

The Cavitron was a marvelous labor-saving device. Dr. Long glanced at the meter on the machine's console. It had actually been on less than an hour, but it had saved him four, maybe five hours of debulking. The thing was heavy, though.

Dr. Long massaged his fingers until the feeling returned. With his right hand as tired as it was, he certainly wouldn't like to be starting in on the basilar right now. As he massaged, he watched the resident's progress on the television monitor. The tag of tumor that he had been assigned to remove was beginning to come free.

Dr. Long considered the neurosurgeons he trained to be his most important contribution to medicine. This resident would be out there operating in less than a year. He would do well. Dr. Long could tell.

Six minutes after he had stepped away from the microscope, Dr. Long was back again.

He didn't go directly to the brain stem, but spent several minutes first cleaning up a bit of tumor material from a less critical area on one side of the hole. Then, satisfied that his hands would obey orders again, he moved his attention back to the brain stem.

Whittle, probe, nudge, tease, coax, urge. The tumor hung on tenaciously, giving ground millimeter by reluctant millimeter.

"It's only hanging on by its teeth," Dr. Long commented.

Coax, tease, urge. Irrigation, please.

A few minutes later, the tumor still firmly in place, Dr. Long amended his earlier statement.

"It's hanging on by its teeth but . . . its teeth are pretty formidable."

Minutes passed, a half hour, an hour.

The chief resident stood back for a time, stretching and watching the television monitor, shifting back and forth from one foot to the other.

The circulating nurse, seated on a stool in a corner, silently assembled a chain of paper clips. Finally the shifts changed, and another nurse took her place. Dr. Long paused momentarily to allow the scrub nurse to brief his replacement. Then the operation resumed.

"We're getting it now, we're getting it now," Dr. Long said suddenly, elation in his voice. "Look. You can see all the edges starting to come out."

It was only starting to come out. That was much different from being out. More minutes passed. The largest remaining chunk of the tumor heaved across the monitor, fell back, heaved again. Finally, it came free.

Out of the head, it looked much smaller, no larger than a nickel.

"Well," said Dr. Long, grinning down at it. "Well, for the first time today, I'm certain that we can cure this boy."

Then he was back at the microscope. Six o'clock came and went.

The brain stem free, Dr. Long turned his attention from the problems that could kill Joe and focused on the problems that could only maim him.

The seventh nerve, for instance, was still partially surrounded by tumor.

Cavitron, please.

Suction.

Irrigation.

Microdissector.

The scrub nurse's hands hovered confidently above the tools, reaching each one as soon as Dr. Long called for it, replacing each one exactly where it belonged.

The stakes were lower, now, but they were still high enough to preserve the tension. Patiently, Dr. Long separated the seventh nerve out of the remaining tumor. Since Joe was apparently going to go back to college, he would need those nerves. They controlled facial muscles, and were absolutely critical for smiling at girls.

Finally, the nerve was free. Now, there was only one remaining speck of tumor—the piece on the jugular bulb.

The microscope focused on the red, blood-filled bag. The instruments reached out, testing the tumor. Nudging, caressing, worrying. Finally, the last piece of yellow tissue was gone.

"By golly," Dr. Long exulted, "that's IT!"

He looked around the operating room, then back into the microscope.

Clean up now, retreat.

First, he took a few minutes to scan the topography. He readjusted the microscope several times. His eyes probed for any speck of yellow, any speck that would grow back into another tumor. But he saw nothing.

He contemplated the landscape in the center of Joe's head. The cranial nerves lay limply across the floor of the cranium, but they were all intact. Some of them might take months to regenerate, but regenerate they would. Joe Trott would live a normal life. It was almost a miracle . . . but not quite.

At 7:22 P.M., Dr. Long stepped back.

"All I've got to say," he groaned, "is that I hope we never see its like again."

As the chief resident moved the microscope out of the way and prepared to close the incision, Dr. Long pulled the rubber gloves from his aching hands and stripped off the bloody surgical cloak.

For a moment he stood, stretching. Then he left the operating room and walked stiffly down the hallway toward the lounge where Joe's parents were waiting. The automatic doors hissed open in front of him.

CHAPTER
TWENTY-SIX

ONCE GEORGE SAMARAS PLUGGED CAPRICORN INTO AN OUTLET BEYOND the walls of the operating room, his brainchild worked perfectly. Carefully, the operating room team and the engineers connected the lead wires to the antenna that protruded from Tony Mastrostephano's head, and then they ran through another series of tests. Perfect. Perfect.

The bioengineers were ready.

The anesthesiologist injected an antidote into the patient's IV line and, a few moments later, Tony moved weakly.

"Tony," Dr. Salcman said, loudly. "Tony! Do you hear me?"

Tony groaned. Yes.

Kay Donnelly, the circulating nurse, stood on her tiptoes to see over Dr. Salcman's shoulder. "How're you doing, Tony?" she asked.

"Well, my head hurts," he answered thickly.

"No kidding," said Kay.

"My head hurts," he groaned again, "but that's all right."

"We're testing the antenna now," Dr. Salcman said.

"Okay. I'm okay. You go ahead and do whatever you need to do."

For precisely fifteen minutes, Capricorn kept the microwave antenna at a constant temperature of one hundred and thirteen Fahrenheit, right on the button, perfect, and then it shut itself off. Until then, Dr. Samaras didn't have to do a thing.

Once the test treatment was finished, Dr. Salcman and the resident moved around to look over Dr. Samaras' shoulder, their eyes on the temperature readouts.

If the probe had heated the cancerous tissue, as it was supposed to, the temperature would fall rapidly as the blood flow carried away the heat. But if it had only heated the liquid around the probe, it would fall more slowly . . . that would not be a good sign.

The numbers fell rapidly, exactly according to theory.

The medical team disconnected Tony from the Capricorn wires, transferred him to a bed and rolled him off toward the CAT-scan room. Dr. Salcman followed.

A half hour later, the neurosurgeon stood in front of the scanner screen, watching the slices assemble themselves in front of him. As he watched the developing images, he couldn't believe his luck.

The antenna was made of soft metal, and it had bent slightly during the insertion. Because of that bend, the heat would be focused on that one remaining piece of visible tumor.

The engineers, in the meantime, went to lunch. As they ate, they puzzled out where the fail-safe, error-checking computer had gone wrong and why it had complained about having no electricity.

The engineers ruefully admitted to one another that they had failed to anticipate one problem, had taken one thing for granted. They had trusted the electricity.

And why not?

Everywhere in the country, in laboratories and residential kitchens, the electricity was the same. A grounded, three-hole receptacle, the safest kind to use and the kind engineers always insisted on, could always be trusted. Two prongs of a three-pronged plug were for tapping the electricity, and the third prong was the ground. The ground made certain a fuse would blow if the circuit became overloaded, or something went wrong.

That was true all over the country . . . except, apparently, in Dr. Salcman's operating room. There, the third wire had not been connected. There was no ground.

Capricorn had been programmed to use the ground wire to check its systems . . . but the engineers had not programmed in a message for it to display if the ground was nonexistent. So the thing didn't know what to say, when it sampled the electricity and found it lacking.

It had responded, in dumb computer fashion, with the message that it had no electricity. The statement was not true, strictly speaking, but it was as close as Capricorn could get.

The fail-safe, error-checking computer had in fact worked as advertised, which was perfectly. It had been the engineers who had been amiss.

Later, talking to the hospital electricians, they would discover why there is no ground in the operating room: Operating rooms are the only exceptions to the rule about grounded electricity. Surgeons didn't *want* a fuse to blow in the operating room, no matter what. If a fuse blew, the respirator would stop. So operating rooms were designed with a set of overload alarm bells, instead.

In the future, an extension cord would have to be part of Capricorn's auxiliary equipment.

As soon as lunch was finished, the engineers went back upstairs. They rolled Capricorn out of the operating room and took it, via elevator, up to the neurosurgical intensive care ward on the twelfth floor. The first thing they did was plug it in, to see if it worked. It did. Perfectly.

A few minutes later Tony was rolled into the room and attached to the monitors. He smiled at the nurses and tried to co-operate with them, but movement was painful. His head still hurt, he said.

"That's okay though," he added. "Don't worry about me. I'm going to be fine."

Before beginning the first full-scale treatment, the medical and engineering teams gathered in a classroom near the intensive care unit. The postoperative CAT scans hung on a lightboard.

Dr. Salcman's eyes were bright with excitement as he explained the various features in the scan films.

For purposes of comparison, he pointed to an earlier scan, taken before the operation, in which the tumor appeared as an elongated white cloud in the forward part of the head. On the postoperative films, there was only one little smudge of white left. That was the bit of tumor that Dr. Salcman had been afraid to take.

And look, he said, at the antenna.

He indicated the long, thin shadow that ran from the outside of the skull to the center of where the tumor used to be. Notice, he said, the slight bend. And notice where the bend would focus the heat.

Luck.

A neurosurgeon isn't supposed to believe in luck. Only skill. Yet, sometimes, the luck runs bad, or good, and a patient's course seems to be more under the influence of the gods than the doctors.

Dr. Salcman looked for a long time at the CAT scan and at the way the temperature probe pointed directly at the remaining bit of tumor.

Tony Mastrostephano would die, of course.

Glioblastoma multiforme patients always died.

But . . .

Luck.

There had to be a first time. There had been a first time for leukemia, a first time for Hodgkin's disease, a first time, even, for lung cancer. There had to be a first time for Glioblastoma multiforme as well. If Dr. Salcman hadn't believed that, hadn't nourished that thin thread of hope . . .

The room was silent, every mind thinking the same thought, rejecting it, then thinking it again.

A few minutes later they filed out of the classroom, and Dr. Salcman made a detour to the lounge. Jean saw him coming, and stubbed out a cigarette. They talked for a minute, or perhaps two. He made her no promises, but she could feel his excitement. After he left she sat, thinking, for a long time, before lighting another cigarette.

When the neurosurgeon arrived in the intensive care cubicle Tony was lying quietly, his eyes closed. The leads had already been connected to the antenna that protruded from the top of his turban of bandages. George Samaras was sitting beside Capricorn.

Dr. Salcman stood above him a moment, watching.

Okay? he asked.

Not "okay." Perfect.

Dr. Salcman walked over to Tony. At the doctor's soft touch on his skin, the patient smiled, but didn't open his eyes. Light made the headache worse.

"Tony?"

"Yes?"

"Tony, we just came back from the operating room. We've got your CAT scan, and it's very good. We got virtually all the tumor out. We're going to start heating the rest again right now."

Tony Mastrostephano took a deep breath. Tears leaked from beneath his tightly-closed eyelids.

Tony's hand groped along the bed rail for Dr. Salcman's, found it, and squeezed it in gratitude. His voice was a faint, trembling whisper.

"We're gonna whip this thing, doc, we're gonna whip it."

Dr. Salcman squeezed Tony's hand.

A few feet away, Dr. Samaras checked the machine one last time, and touched a button. Soon there was a faint hum. Numbers flashed on the readouts. Time and temperature readings flickered across the computer screen.

Perfect.

Absolutely perfect.

CHAPTER
TWENTY-SEVEN

Dr. Ducker stood in front of the X-ray board in Operating Room Eleven, his gloved hands held close against his sterile gown. Time after time, he had come to the X-ray board to stand and stare, his mind analyzing, memorizing, visualizing the tentacled monster he was about to face. Every secret must be wrung from the films, every hint, every bit of conscious and subconscious intelligence.

For days, he had devoted an increasing amount of time to the study of Richard's films. He had discussed them with the neuro-radiologist, and again, several times, with the neurologists. He didn't want to miss a thing.

In his view an arteriovenous malformation was one of the craftiest enemies a neurosurgeon could face, and he approached them with extreme trepidation.

In one sense, removing an AVM was a relatively straightforward process. The monster didn't invade normal brain tissue like a cancer —nor did it stick to everything like an acoustic tumor.

The danger of an AVM was simple, very simple indeed. The danger of an AVM was Big Red.

The body of the monster would be a large, thin pouch the size of a walnut. A network of tentacles would be coming off from the bag— the enlarged veins that had been developed to carry away all the blood.

The challenge would be to find exactly where the bag was being fed by an artery or arteries. Richard's AVM, according to the X-rays, had two different feeders. Once they were clipped, pressure would fall inside the bag, and the monster, tentacles and all, could be removed.

The danger would come as he tried to clip the arteries. He couldn't do that without disturbing the bag, and it must be very fragile. It had bled once already, without even being touched.

For that matter, the AVM might explode as soon as he opened the skull. That happened, sometimes. Blooey, and the wolf was at the door: Then there was no way you could be ready for it, no way you could get to the center of the brain fast enough.

Once he got the bag clipped, the rest would be routine.

In the meantime, he wanted to know as much as he could possibly know about where everything was in relation to everything else.

Dr. Ducker gazed at the films. Behind him, Richard lay on the operating table, unconscious, a plastic respirator tube protruding from his mouth. A resident scrubbed brown antiseptic onto his shaved head.

Dr. Ducker studied, for perhaps the hundredth time, the white fuzzy blob that sat right above the Circle of Willis.

The Circle of Willis was a ring of arteries that lay on the bony floor of the forebrain, right between the ears. All the huge quantities of blood that supplied the upper brain rose through the Circle of Willis, which made it a frightening place to work.

Navigation would be critically important. The bag was nestled in the center of the Sylvian Triangle, the area between the circle and its two foremost arteries, the anterior and middle cerebrals. The films showed large feeder vessels leading to the AVM from both arteries.

Dr. Ducker stared at the X-rays. To get there, he would have to pry the brain apart, lift the frontal lobe, push the temporal lobe aside, and dive into the brain at a forty-five-degree angle, sticking where he could to natural separations between lobes, until he had created a long, narrow tunnel with the monster at the end of it. Then he would have to reach down, with clips . . .

Thoughtfully, the neurosurgeon turned away from the X-ray board. The steady beep, beep, beep of the heart monitor was reassuring to his ears.

Once again, he reviewed his fallback positions.

The residents had begun placing sterile drapes on the patient and the anesthesiologist stood by to protect his tubes and cords. Within a few minutes, all that was visible of Richard was a window of scalp that ran from above his eyebrows across the right side of his head.

Watching the residents work, Dr. Ducker chuckled to himself. He'd spent the morning doing squirrels. In one respect, it was harder to do squirrels than people. He had residents to open up people for him . . . but he had to open his own squirrels. Life was funny.

"Anesthesia okay?" he asked.

"Fine," the anesthesiologist replied. The lights glowed on the computerized monitors, and the readings were stable. Blood pressure one twenty-two over eighty-two, pulse seventy-six, steady.

Dr. Ducker walked over to the patient, took a sterile marking pencil and traced the incision he wanted the resident to make in Richard's scalp. The line began just above the right ear, rose to the top of the head and curved down toward the center of the forehead. It stopped right at the hairline; Dr. Ducker hated to make scars on people's faces.

Dr. Ducker stepped back to supervise, and the resident called for a scalpel. He pushed hard on the blade, driving it all the way to the skull. Blood welled up, and scalp clips snapped into place.

By the time the resident had finished the incision, stopped the bleeding, and scraped the scalp flap off the skull with a chisel, it was 12:48 P.M.

The heart monitor beeped steadily, seventy-six beats a minute.

The anesthesiologist kept the blood pressure down, just in case. She had also given the patient a drug, mannitol, that increased urine output. That caused the body to lose liquid and shrink. The brain, shrunken a little, would be easier to push aside.

"Craniotome," the resident said.

He pressed the bit against Richard's skull. The piercing zhoop-zhoop ZHOOOOOOOOOOOOOOOOOOOOOOOO filled the operating room. Powdered bone piled up around the holes. Soon there were four holes, one at each corner of the planned bone flap.

Dr. Ducker helped the resident thread the rough wire bone saw in one hole and out the other, then stood back as the younger man pulled the wire back and forth until the holes were connected by a narrow slit. After the process had been completed four times, the bone flap lifted free.

With a smaller bit in the craniotome, the neurosurgeons drilled matching holes in the bone flap and the surrounding skull, so the bone could be wired into place at the end of the operation. Then the scrub nurse wrapped the piece of bone in wet gauze pads, put it in a small metal bowl, and set it aside.

At 1:26 the resident opened the dura and peeled it back from the brain. The gray surface glistened in the surgical spotlight.

The abnormality was obvious, even to the scrub nurse. Three large, red vessels rose from individual crevices and extended, narrowing, across the convolutions of the brain.

Tentacles.

Dr. Ducker stooped close to examine one of them.

"They're enlarged veins," he said. "See how red they are?"

Venous blood, depleted of oxygen, was blue. Only arterial blood was red.

"That vein's draining the AVM."

Dr. Ducker straightened up, tucked his hands in close to his chest, and walked again to the X-ray board. He studied how the tentacles dove through the brain, growing ever larger, until they reached the AVM. In a moment, he returned to the operating lights.

"We'll go through the cortex right here," he said to the resident, pointing at the spot where the largest of the red veins disappeared into the Sylvian fissure.

The operating microscope swung into place. By 1:45 P.M. the room was dark, except for the 'scope's tiny bright headlight.

The resident examined the landscape while adjusting the focus. Under fifteen magnifications, the red vein throbbed and danced in time to the beeping of the heart monitor, seventy-six beats a minute, seventy-six beats a minute, steady, unchanging, stable.

A door opened slightly and two medical students slipped through. Saying nothing, making no noise, they moved immediately to a corner of the OR that had an unobstructed view of the television monitor screen.

The titanium instruments, smaller than a watchmaker's tools, loomed huge on the screen. Moving slowly and awkwardly under the magnification, they probed at the Sylvian fissure, near where the tentacle disappeared into it.

The inner membrane, the pia, dove into the fissure, following the finest contours of the brain. But the middle membrane, the arachnoid, leaped across it and barred the surgical advance. It had to be carefully nudged and poked until it parted.

Underneath, gray brain cells throbbed, held back only by the vanishingly thin pia.

The medical students watched the monitor, silently.

A long, thin instrument with a tiny spatula at one end entered the operating field from the right side. From the left there appeared an equally tiny, tweezers-like instrument—the micro-bipolars.

The spatula wriggled into the Sylvian fissure, next to the tentacle, and pried.

No, not pried.

Slowly, very slowly, the fissure parted. Helped by the mannitol, the sides seemed to sigh, and draw away.

The spatula moved a fraction of a centimeter, inserted itself, and coaxed again. The bipolars lingered nearby, in case . . . always in case.

The minutes passed and the heart monitor beeped steadily, seventy-six beats a minute.

Patiently the tools worked their way deeper, deeper, a millimeter at a time. Long, narrow retractors moved into the field and gently, gently, were fixed in place, shoring up the sides of the tunnel.

The tunnel led downward and downward, following the tentacle. At the sides, the gray jelly of the brain heaved and throbbed behind the delicate, transparent pia. The instruments took care never to touch the pia unnecessarily.

Once, a tiny blood vessel broke under the pressure. A red stream fountained up, squirting with the heart monitor, seventy-six times a minute. Blood crept across the field.

"Irrigation," the resident said.

Sterile water swirled across the field, diluting the blood and then disappearing up the barrel of a suction probe.

Then, the field clear, the bipolars moved into view, hesitated, and pounced on the spurting artery. Sparks flew between the tips of the bipolars, once, twice, three times for good measure.

Cautiously, the bipolars moved back a little bit, hesitantly, ready to jump forward. But there was no renewed bleeding.

The spatula reappeared and worked the tunnel deeper and deeper, millimeter by tortuous millimeter.

"That was about half a cc of blood," Dr. Ducker said, for the benefit of the medical students. "Under this much magnification it looks like a lot more."

They knew they were nearing the AVM when other reddish tentacles began converging in the tunnel. They were large, this near the monster. Large . . . and fragile.

The resident backed away from the main 'scope. Dr. Ducker took his place.

It was 1:56.

Gently, slowly, Dr. Ducker worked around the tentacles, pushing the tunnel deeper, urging the temporal lobe slightly to the side, coaxing the frontal lobe up ever so slightly, deeper, deeper toward the center of the brain.

With increasing depth, the long-handled tools became more difficult to control. Each millimeter grew more dangerous, more costly in terms of surgical energy. And now, increasingly, there was blood in the field. It was bright-red blood, but it didn't come from a bleeder, and it didn't spurt. It was the monster itself. It was leaking.

Irrigation.

Again.

Suction.

Irrigation.

Move forward a millimeter.

Irrigation.

Suction.

The heart beat steady, seventy-six beats a minute.

Suddenly the thing loomed large in the microscopic field, a tangle of bulging, pulsing, reddish ropelike veins. The AVM. The monster.

"There it is. That's what we're here for. I need a clip, please," Dr. Ducker said in a quiet voice.

It was 2:05.

Dr. Ducker examined his foe through the microscope. The bag was in the background, behind the tentacles.

Of the two feeders, the more distant one would be the more difficult to clip. To get at it, he'd have to reach around, gently, and urge the bag aside, and find the feeder, and then maneuver a clip over it.

The one in front would be easy, by comparison. He'd do the difficult one first.

The scrub nurse picked up a spring-loaded clip and fastened it in an instrument that held its long, thin jaws open. She handed the loaded instrument to the surgeon.

Gingerly, he lowered it into the surgical wound, deep into Richard's brain, until it appeared in the microscopic field. Soon it was joined by a probe that gently urged the monster aside. Far in the background, the feeder throbbed with pressure.

The clip approached the feeder, hesitated, and turned slightly. It moved to one side, as though examining the situation, and approached again.

Dr. Ducker frowned into the microscope and withdrew the instrument.

"I need a larger clip," he said.

As the nurse loaded it, the neurosurgeon continued to stare down the microscope barrels. When she was ready, he reached out a hand and she put the instrument into it. The resident helped guide the clip-holder toward the hole.

The larger clip now approached, turned, hesitated, approached, turned and stopped. Then it moved forward, slowly, steadily, until its jaws were over the feeder.

Dr. Ducker touched a trigger at the top of the instrument and the jaws snapped closed.

"That's clipped," he said.

One down, one to go.

Retreating a short distance down the surgical tunnel, Dr. Ducker let the monster settle back down over the clipped feeder. Nothing happened.

He withdrew the instruments and stepped back, then readjusted the microscope for the second approach. He squinted into the eyepieces.

A metal probe moved across the field, separating the tangle of tentacles in front. Finally, the monster's second neck, this one a branch off the middle cerebral artery, was in view.

"Okay, let's have another clip."

The scrub nurse laid the instrument in his hand.

The clip appeared on the monitor screen, hesitated, and moved toward the feeder. The medical students watched the television monitor.

The clip moved, and its jaws snapped down on the feeder.

The pressure relieved, the bag sagged slightly.

Dr. Ducker stepped back.

"Well," he said to the medical students. "That's the hard part. Now let's do the easy part."

It was 2:15.

"Microscissors," he said.

The scissors appeared in the field, followed by the ever present bipolars. The bipolars moved forward, poked at one of the tentacles and gently tugged it free. The scissors maneuvered for position, then closed over the tentacle and snipped it.

A gush of blood instantly swirled across the field, submerging the monster and its tentacles in a rising crimson lake.

Dr. Ducker stared down the barrels of the microscope, dumbfounded.

Then he reacted.

"Suction."

The words were soft, even, carefully measured.

The nurse placed the sucker in his right hand, and helped the resident arrange the plastic hose across the drapes. Then she hurried to get a second suction probe ready.

"And turn up the vacuum a little," instructed Dr. Ducker as he lowered the sucker into the tunnel.

The blood level, in the meantime, had been rising up through the tunnel. Dr. Ducker lowered the suction tip into the lake of blood. The sucker made a whirlpool in the blood, and the level stopped rising . . . but it didn't fall.

As he waited for the second sucker, Dr. Ducker's mind raced. There hadn't been two feeders, there must have been three. The X-rays had betrayed him.

He would have to find that third one, and clip it, fast.

The heart still beat steady, seventy-six beats a minute.

Soon a second sucker was lowered into the red lake, and the level began to drop. But the landscape that rose above the lake was still red with blood, and seeing was difficult.

"Irrigation."

The water washed away the blood and raised the level of the lake. Slowly, it dropped again.

With the two suckers controlling the depth of the lake, Dr. Ducker took the spatula and began, as quickly as he dared, to push up over the top of the monster.

Where was the feeder? Where was the damned feeder?

"Irrigation."

He saw nothing. He pushed farther.

On the other side of the operating table, the anesthesiologist had sensed the sudden tension in the air and looked up just as the monitor screen had turned blood red.

As Dr. Ducker had fought to drop the level of the red lake, the anesthesiologist had quietly filled a syringe and injected it into Richard's IV line. Now she sat and watched the monitors. The blood pressure faltered, and dropped, and dropped, and dropped, and finally stabilized at a very low eighty over fifty. That should slow the bleeding.

"I took his pressure down," she announced when it had stabilized. "Does that help?"

"Yeah. Thanks," Dr. Ducker said, never moving his eyes from the microscope.

"Irrigation."

The lowered blood pressure did help, and the lake went down some more.

Suddenly, Dr. Ducker saw an image in the background. He lost it, then found it again, a throbbing feeder behind a veil of tentacles. He lost it again.

"Clip," he said.

The scrub nurse had it ready. She slapped it into his hand.

He lost it, found it, lost it.

"Irrigation."

It moved, there, in the background. The clip moved toward it, but hesitated.

Too much blood. Hard to see.

"Irrigation."

Beep, beep, beep, beep . . .

He had time, but not much, now.

There it was.

The students didn't see the feeder, but they saw the clip suddenly plunge into the red landscape, and snap. For a moment it was visible, shining in the microscope's headlight, then the tentacles settled over it.

The lake fell now, rapidly. There were still bleeders, but they were small, secondary ones. They could be handled by the bipolars.

"Irrigation."

The swirling water washed away the blood, and for a moment, a distant metal clip glittered.

The bipolars moved, and electricity crackled.

The bipolars withdrew, and hovered.

"Irrigation."

The bipolars hesitated, then grabbed.

Zzzzzt.

And moved on.

"Irrigation."

Zzzzzzt.

With each new vein cauterized, the blood flow lessened. Finally, it stopped completely.

"What's his pressure?" the neurosurgeon asked the anesthesiologist.

"Fifty-five."

"You can run it up a little bit, now. We're under control."

Dr. Ducker stood, flexed his shoulders, and breathed deeply. The heart monitor beeped steadily, seventy-six beats a minute, seventy-six beats a minute.

Then he stepped to the microscope again, and the bipolars swam into view on the monitor.

The monster now defused, the bipolars found the first clip and burned the vessel shut behind it. Then the second, then the third. The smell of burned flesh was strong.

With the increase in pressure, several more small bleeders broke loose in the field.

Irrigation.

Suction.

Zzzzzt.

Irrigation.

It was 2:21.

"What y'all just saw," Dr. Ducker said, raising his voice for the benefit of the medical students, "was something that shouldn't have happened. We thought we had it clipped, but it fooled us. The X-rays said there were two feeders. There were three. I found that out the hard way. It cost us about half a pint of blood."

"Now we've got that under control, and we'll go ahead and take the AVM out."

The now flaccid bag of veins came loose from the surrounding brain tissue easily. Dr. Ducker worked his way slowly along the monster's arterial connections, clipping them one at a time with the microscissors, then teasing them free.

As he did, he kept up a running commentary for the resident and medical students, using the bipolars to point out the original neck of the AVM and the hidden feeder behind it.

He worked his way around the deflated monster, and methodically freed it from its tentacles and other connections.

The monster came out in chunks, small ones first, then larger and larger ones. Finally, Dr. Ducker reached in with the tweezers and withdrew a large white mass that looked like a tangle of half-cooked spaghetti. The scrub nurse extended a metal bowl and the monster plopped softly into it.

"How about that," Dr. Ducker said. "That's it."

He backed away from the microscope. The resident moved in to begin the closure. Dr. Ducker helped push the microscope out of the way and then stood behind the resident, to watch him work.

Dr. Ducker glanced at the clock.

It was only 3:10.

There was plenty of time for rounds.

EPILOGUE

AFTER A SUCCESSFUL BRAIN OPERATION, THE RELATIONSHIP BETWEEN patient and doctor gradually loses its intensity. Several days after Richard's operation, he returned home to his wife and new baby girl. Four weeks after that, he was back at work at the Mental Health Center. Periodically, Dr. Ducker saw him at the clinic, but he didn't wake up at night thinking about him. As for Richard, he had no further need for Dr. Ducker in his life.

Likewise, the less Joe Trott saw of doctors and hospitals, the better . . . though for several months, he had little choice. Slowly, he got better. As his cranial nerves recovered, he regained his ability to swallow without inhaling and was allowed to eat solid food. Each day, more physical therapy. He was better, he thought. A lot better.

School?

Not yet, they told him, as he chafed at the endless recuperation. Six weeks in the hospital! He didn't have time for that nonsense!

He was in a hurry to get back, but when the day finally came . . . nothing was the same.

The buildings were still there, of course. And the stadium. And the teachers. But they were somehow altered.

It was all very serious now. There was no time for firecrackers, or practical jokes. Anmar . . . Anmar really needed to be retired. The time for Anmar was over. Life was short, too short to waste playing Dungeons and Dragons.

At the end of the first quarter, his name appeared, for the first time, on the dean's list.

Tony, a few weeks after his last treatment with Capricorn, went home to eat lobster tails, recover his strength and swim in his neighbor's pool. In that fashion, the summer passed and the headaches did not return.

"I'm going to lick this thing," he told his friends.

And, with Jean by his side, he waited. Periodically, he came to Baltimore to see Dr. Salcman.

A year after the operation, the headaches still had not returned. Other things occupied his mind, now. Computers. Football. Lobsters.

Jean.

The relationship between neurosurgeon and patient lapses, as both move on to other things, other problems, other challenges. Dr. Salcman's transphenoidal patient and her family returned to their home in South America. Dr. Salcman heard from a relative that the girl continued to improve, and was recovering her former beauty. With luck, she would never see Dr. Salcman again.

But sometimes there is a final, extra gesture.

Dr. Ducker stood looking down at Josh Machat. The boy wiggled his hand.

First base, huh?

Yes, sir.

You ever hear of a fellow named Doug DeCinces?

Sure. Doug DeCinces was the Orioles' brilliant third baseman.

Dr. Ducker had an idea. The next time Josh was due to come in for an examination, he promised, they would do something special.

There were certain privileges to being a prominent neurosurgeon. Doug DeCinces was one of his patients.

The appointed day dawned gray and chilly, and the rain came down in torrents. Occasionally, Dr. Ducker looked out the window. Damn. Something can always happen.

But sometimes, there is luck.

The rain broke a half hour before the game. The sun moved out from behind the clouds, and made Memorial Stadium's asphalt parking lot shimmer and gleam.

Josh Machat jumped out of the car. His parents emerged more cautiously, looking at the sky. But the chill was suddenly gone.

Josh wore an Orioles baseball cap and an orange plastic batter's cap over that. His healing left hand was concealed by a big first baseman's mitt.

"C'mon," he said. Parents are slow.

They were early. As they walked toward the stadium, the parking lot slowly filled with cars. Soon Barbara Ducker and the three Ducker children arrived, along with Barbara Burns, Dr. Ducker's secretary. Finally, a few minutes before the game, Dr. Ducker himself drove up. He spotted the group from a hundred yards away, and waved.

He took Josh by the hand and they all went inside. For a few minutes, they all waited in the hall. Then Doug DeCinces emerged from
an unmarked door.

"Doug, this is Josh," Dr. Ducker said.

Josh craned his neck upward. The bill of his batter's cap came to
slightly below the third baseman's belt.

The baseball player squatted down and held out his hand. Josh's
hand disappeared into it.

"Well, Josh, I hear you can play baseball again."

Josh nodded solemnly.

"What do you play?"

Josh looked at the floor. "First base," he whispered.

Grinning, DeCinces stood up. "C'mon, Josh. Let's see if we can find
a baseball to sign for you."

The boy followed the third baseman back through the door.

A few minutes later, Josh emerged clutching a signature-covered
baseball. His mother said something about a glass case. She took the
ball for safekeeping, and put it in her purse.

Josh didn't say anything. His eyes were on the door behind which
Doug DeCinces was getting ready to go out and play baseball.

The group wound up the ramps and found their way to the seats
that the third baseman had reserved in Dr. Ducker's name. Once everybody was settled, Dr. Ducker asked Josh to show him his left hand.

Josh carefully took off his jacket, rolled up his left shirt sleeve and
presented his outstretched arm to Dr. Ducker. The neurosurgeon
solemnly examined it, noting the thin, neat scar, testing with a fingertip to see how much sensation had returned.

"I think he's going to be fine," he told Josh's parents.

The sun shone down on the wet seats, and the sparkling outfield,
and the Orioles. By the end of the first inning, Baltimore led Cleve-
land, 4 to 1.

Josh sat still for a while, then got restless. The truth was, he'd rather
play than watch.

Along with the Ducker boys, Josh wandered around the stadium,
mesmerized by the sights and sounds. Later he returned, crawled into
his mother's lap and sat contentedly, leafing through the official program.

"I saw him in the locker room," he told Dr. Ducker, pointing to a
picture of Al Bumbry.

But, in the bottom of the third, when Doug DeCinces walked
calmly up to the plate, Josh paid attention.

The third baseman swung his bat experimentally twice, then hunched over into a batting stance.

Josh watched, spellbound.

Len Barker, the Indians' pitcher, fired a fast ball.

DeCinces stepped back. The ball smacked into the catcher's mitt.

Outside, the umpire motioned. Ball one.

Josh stared, silent, waiting, both fists clenched on the pipe railing in front of him.

DeCinces tapped the plate with his bat.

The pitcher wound up and threw.

Another fast ball.

DeCinces swung hard. The solid *crack* of bat hitting ball echoed off the stadium walls.

For an instant, DeCinces stood still.

The ball rose sharply into the clear blue sky, reached the top of its arc, and fell, slowly at first, then steeply, just inside the third base line. In the stands, hands reached up for the home-run ball.

As DeCinces trotted around the bases Josh jumped up and down and screamed triumphantly.

INDEX

Acid, drug addiction and, 54
Acoustic nerve tumor (acoustic
   neurinoma), 8, 41–49, 79, 90–99,
   101–3, 111–12, 115–25, 159–69,
   225–45, 261; described, kinds,
   size and symptoms of, 41–49,
   115, 227, 242; postoperative care
   and, 159–69, 171–78; surgery
   for, 91, 93–99, 101–3, 111–12,
   115–25
Albuquerque, Edson, 132, 134, 135
Alcoholism, 61
American College of
   Neurosurgeons, 72
Amphetamines (speed, uppers),
   28, 54, 55
Anatomy. See Neuroanatomy;
   specific body parts, surgical
   procedures
Anesthesiologists, surgery and, 13,
   14, 16, 40, 247; acoustic nerve
   tumor surgery and, 93, 99, 117,
   166, 225–26, 230, 241; AVM
   surgery and, 253, 258–59;
   glioblastoma multiforme surgery
   and, 214, 221; pituitary tumor
   surgery and, 66, 72, 81; ulnar
   nerve surgery and, 13, 14, 16, 40
Aneurysms, 31, 39, 91, 121, 143,
   179
Anger, neurotransmitters and, 29
Angioblastoma, 91
Angiogram, 116, 181
Antacids, use of, 162
Anterior inferior cerebellar artery
   (AICA, aye-ka), 98, 102–3, 115,
116, 118, 122, 124, 229, 232, 236,
   240, 242, 243
Antibiotics, use of, 161, 162, 167,
   168, 176
Anticonvulsants, 166, 167, 168
Arachnoid (arachnoid
   membrane), 24, 99, 102, 165;
   acoustic nerve tumor surgery
   and, 99, 102, 165; AVM surgery
   and, 254
Association for Brain Tumor
   Research, 183
Astrocytoma, 148–49
Atelectasis, 175
Atherosclerosis, 142
Auditory nerve, 118, 242. See also
   Acoustic nerve tumor; Deafness
AVM (arteriovenous
   malformation), 39, 143, 179–81,
   207–11; surgcial removal of, 180,
   207–11, 251–60
Axons, 17, 29, 30, 31, 135; defined,
   described, 29; ulnar nerve
   surgery and, 17, 35, 37, 38, 39
Aye-ka. See Anterior inferior
   cerebellar artery

Back pain, surgery and, 104, 105,
   200, 202
Bacteria, 27. See also Infections
Balance problems, acoustic nerve
   tumors and, 47
Baltimore, Md. See University of
   Maryland Medical School and
   Hospital
Barrel clips, 95. See also Clips